"Weeknight Vegan & Vegetarian Delights: A Month of Healthy Dinners for Busy Lives"

By Jenny Koo

"Weeknight Vegan & Vegetarian Delights: A Month of Healthy Dinners for Busy Lives"

Introduction

- Welcome
- Benefits of Cooking at Home
- How to Use This Cookbook

Chapter 1: Quick Start Guide

- Kitchen Essentials
- Meal Planning Tips
- Time-Saving Techniques

Chapter 2: Vegan & Vegetarian Basics

- Introduction to Vegan and Vegetarian Cooking
- Essential Ingredients
- Cooking Methods

Chapter 3: Weeknight Dinner Meal Plans

- Week 1
    - Monday: [Recipe]
    - Tuesday: [Recipe]
    - Wednesday: [Recipe]
    - Thursday: [Recipe]
    - Friday: [Recipe]
- Week 2
    - Repeat format for each day
- Week 3
    - Repeat format for each day
- Week 4
    - Repeat format for each day

Chapter 4: Recipes

- Quick and Easy Dinners
    - [Recipe 1]
    - [Recipe 2]

- [Recipe 3]
- One-Pot Wonders
  - [Recipe 4]
  - [Recipe 5]
  - [Recipe 6]
- Sheet Pan Delights
  - [Recipe 7]
  - [Recipe 8]
  - [Recipe 9]
- Flavorful Stir-Fries
  - [Recipe 10]
  - [Recipe 11]
  - [Recipe 12]
- Comforting Soups and Stews
  - [Recipe 13]
  - [Recipe 14]
  - [Recipe 15]
- Nutrient-Packed Bowls
  - [Recipe 16]
  - [Recipe 17]
  - [Recipe 18]

Chapter 5: Leftover Lunch Ideas

- Creative Ways to Repurpose Dinner Leftovers
- Lunchbox-Friendly Recipes

Chapter 6: Bonus Templates

- Weekly Meal Planner
- Shopping List Template
- Recipe Notes

Chapter 7: Tips for Dining Out on Weekends

- Making Healthy Choices
- Restaurant Survival Guide

Conclusion

- Recap of Benefits
- Encouragement for a Healthier Lifestyle

Appendix

- Ingredient Substitution Guide
- Metric Conversion Chart

Encouragement

- Encouragement from the author

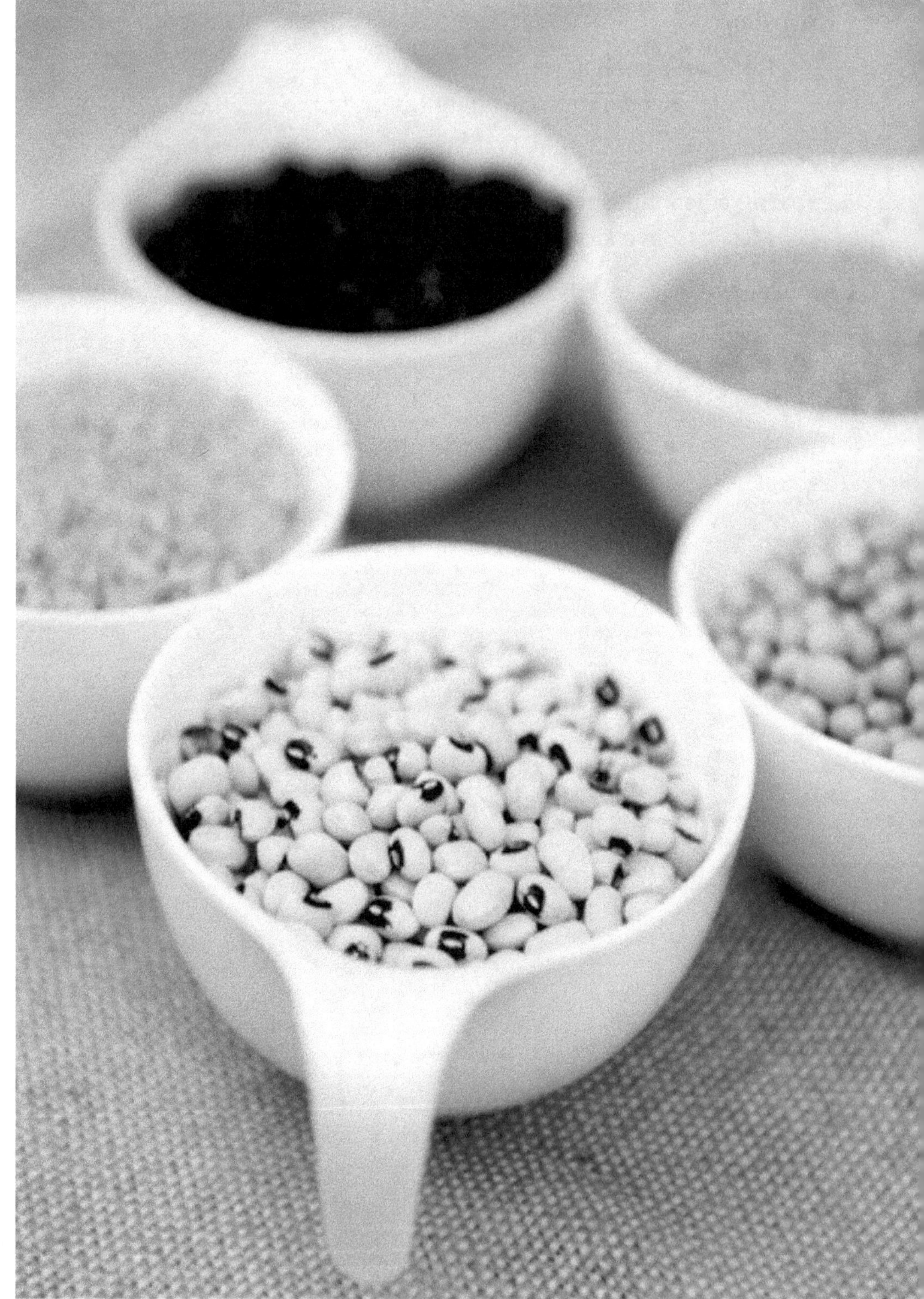

Introduction

- Welcome
- Benefits of Cooking at Home
- How to Use This Cookbook

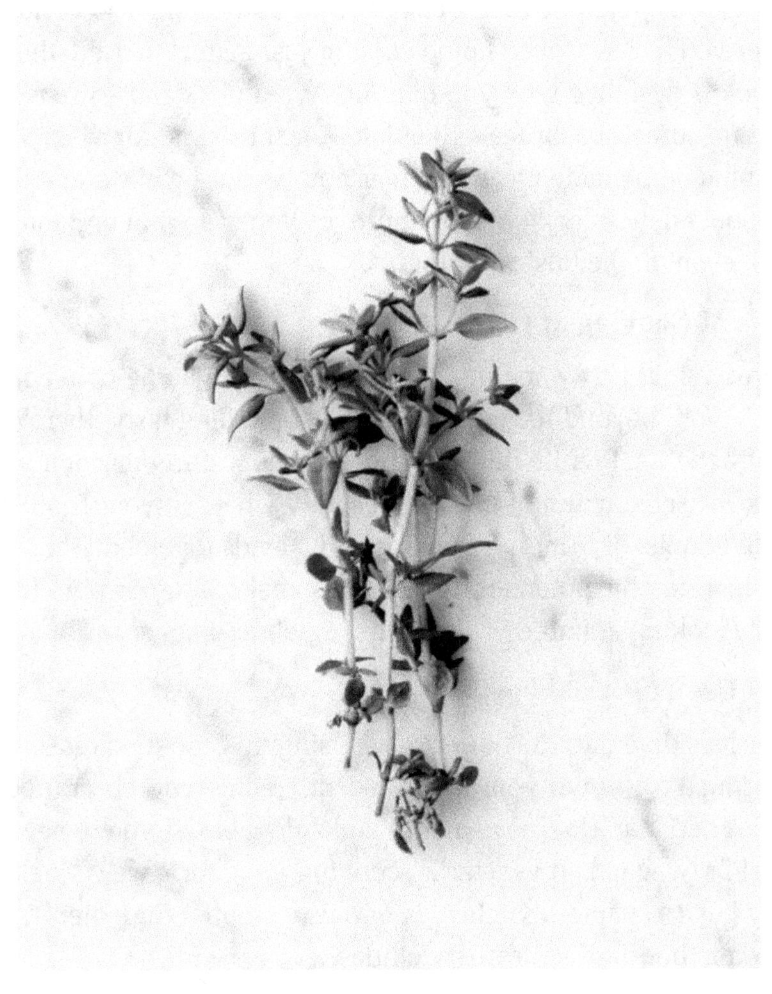

Introduction

Hey there, kitchen adventurer! Welcome to "Weeknight Vegan & Vegetarian Delights," your passport to a month of mouthwatering, healthy dinners crafted specifically for those bustling weeknights.

Welcome

First off, a big welcome to our cozy corner of the culinary world. Whether you're a seasoned home cook or just getting started, this cookbook is designed with you in mind. We understand – life is hectic, and sometimes it feels like there's just no time for a wholesome homemade meal. But fear not, because we're about to embark on a delicious journey that proves you can whip up fantastic dinners, even on the busiest of nights.

Benefits of Cooking at Home

Now, you might be wondering, "Why bother with home-cooked meals?" Well, beyond the joy of creating something tasty, there's a trove of benefits. Picture this: sizzling aromas wafting through your kitchen, the satisfaction of knowing exactly what's in your food, and the added bonus of bringing families and friends together. Oh, and did we mention the potential for leftovers, making tomorrow's lunch a breeze? Cooking at home is like a mini celebration every day!

How to Use This Cookbook

Alright, let's dive into the nitty-gritty. Using this cookbook is as easy as savoring a forkful of your favorite dish. Each section is crafted to make your culinary journey smooth and enjoyable. If you're new to the world of vegan and vegetarian cooking, fear not – we've included a handy basics chapter. Kitchen essentials, essential ingredients, and cooking methods are your trusty guides.

As you flip through the pages, you'll discover weeknight meal plans and quick and easy recipes, each designed to serve a small family of 4 or 5 servings. Plus, there's a thoughtful twist – intentional leftover portions that make for a delightful next-day lunch. Feel free to mix and match, adapt, and make these recipes your own. And if you ever find yourself in a culinary conundrum, our friendly Bonus Templates section has your back with weekly meal planners, shopping lists, and space for jotting down your culinary masterpieces.

So, buckle up, my friend. Your kitchen adventure is about to begin. Let's make weeknight dinners not just a necessity but a delightful experience. Happy cooking!

Chapter 1: Quick Start Guide

- Kitchen Essentials
- Meal Planning Tips
- Time-Saving Techniques

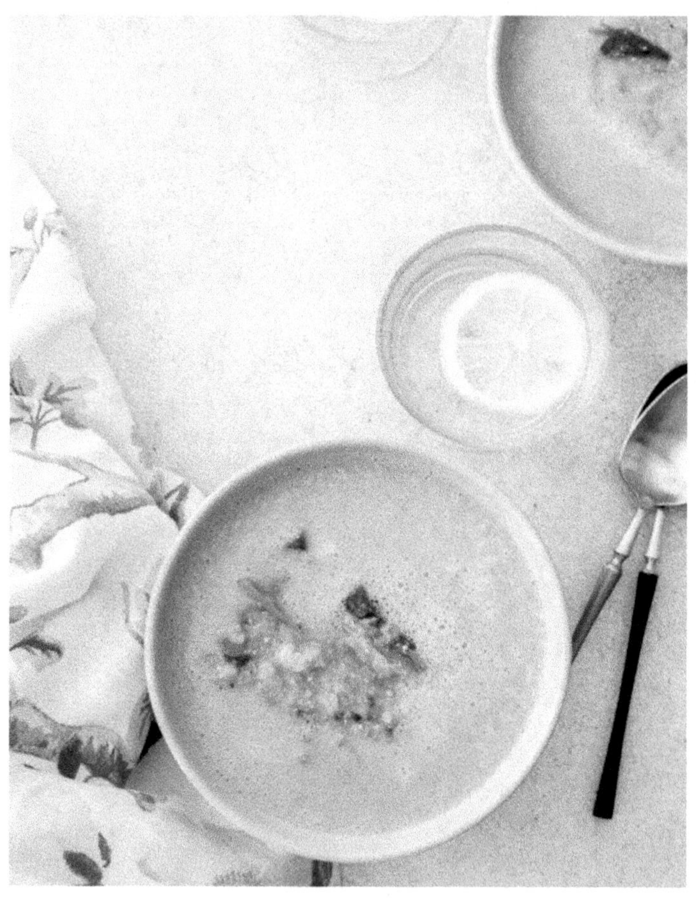

Chapter 1: Quick Start Guide

Welcome to the Quick Start Guide, your gateway to mastering the art of weeknight cooking. This chapter is designed to not only acquaint you with essential kitchen tools but also empower you with efficient meal planning tips and time-saving techniques.

Kitchen Essentials

The Foundation of Your Culinary Haven

In this section, we'll explore the fundamental tools that form the backbone of every well-equipped kitchen. From a high-quality chef's knife to a sturdy cutting board, we'll guide you through selecting tools that are both practical and versatile. Learn about the pots and pans that suit your cooking style, and discover the magic behind certain gadgets that can make your cooking experience more efficient. By the end of this section, you'll feel confident in your kitchen domain, ready to embark on flavorful adventures.

1. **Chef's Knife:** The unsung hero of every kitchen. Invest in a quality chef's knife; it's the workhorse that will make chopping, dicing, and slicing a breeze.

2. **Cutting Board:** Choose a durable, easy-to-clean cutting board. Consider separate boards for veggies and proteins to prevent cross-contamination.

3. **Pots and Pans:** Build your collection with a versatile set, including a saucepan, skillet, and a sturdy pot. These basics cover a wide range of cooking techniques.

4. **Utensils:** A spatula, ladle, and tongs are your kitchen companions. Make sure they're heat-resistant and durable.

5. **Measuring Tools:** Precision matters. Invest in measuring cups and spoons for accurate ingredient quantities.

6. **Gadgets:** While not mandatory, tools like a garlic press, vegetable peeler, and microplane can save time and add finesse to your dishes.

Meal Planning Tips

Strategize Your Culinary Week

Effective meal planning is the secret ingredient to stress-free weeknight dinners. In this part of the guide, we'll delve into the art of planning, helping you organize your culinary week like a pro. Discover how themed nights can add variety without complexity, and learn to leverage ingredient overlap to minimize waste. We'll also discuss the importance of keeping a well-stocked pantry and share tips for adapting recipes to fit your schedule. With our insights, you'll transform meal planning from a chore into a creative and enjoyable process.

1. **Themed Nights:** Simplify your planning by assigning themes to different nights—Mexican Mondays, Pasta Tuesdays, and so on. It adds a fun twist to your routine.

2. **Ingredient Overlap:** Plan meals that share common ingredients. It reduces waste and simplifies your shopping list.

3. **Batch Cooking:** Spend a bit more time on weekends preparing staples like grains, beans, and sauces. It streamlines weeknight cooking and adds variety to your meals.

4. **Freezer-Friendly Meals:** Embrace the freezer. Prepare larger batches and freeze portions for those extra busy nights when cooking from scratch feels challenging.

5. **Flexibility:** Be open to switching days or repurposing leftovers. Flexibility is the key to stress-free meal planning.

Time-Saving Techniques

Efficiency Without Compromise

Time is of the essence on busy weeknights, and this section is your key to unlocking efficiency in the kitchen. Explore time-saving techniques that enhance your cooking experience without sacrificing flavor. From mastering the art of efficient chopping to embracing batch-cooking strategies, you'll learn how to make the most of your precious time. We believe that cooking should be a joy, not a burden, and these techniques will pave the way for more moments of culinary delight and fewer instances of kitchen chaos.

1. **Efficient Chopping:** Master the art of chopping by adopting proper techniques. Practice can significantly reduce your prep time.

2. **One-Pan Wonders:** Opt for recipes that require minimal cleanup. Sheet pan dinners and one-pot wonders are not only time-efficient but also flavorful.

3. **Batch Prep:** Prep ingredients in batches when possible. Chop extra veggies, marinate proteins, or make sauces ahead of time for quick assembly on busy nights.

4. **Simultaneous Cooking:** Learn to multitask in the kitchen. While one element is cooking, use that time to prep or clean up.

5. **Smart Kitchen Organization:** Keep your kitchen organized to avoid unnecessary searches for utensils or ingredients. A well-organized kitchen is a time-saving kitchen.

By the time you finish this Quick Start Guide, you'll not only have a well-stocked kitchen but also a strategic approach to meal planning and time management. So, grab your apron and get ready to turn your kitchen into a haven of delicious possibilities!

Chapter 2: Vegan & Vegetarian Basics

- ⌄ Introduction to Vegan and Vegetarian Cooking
- ⌄ Essential Ingredients
- ⌄ Cooking Methods

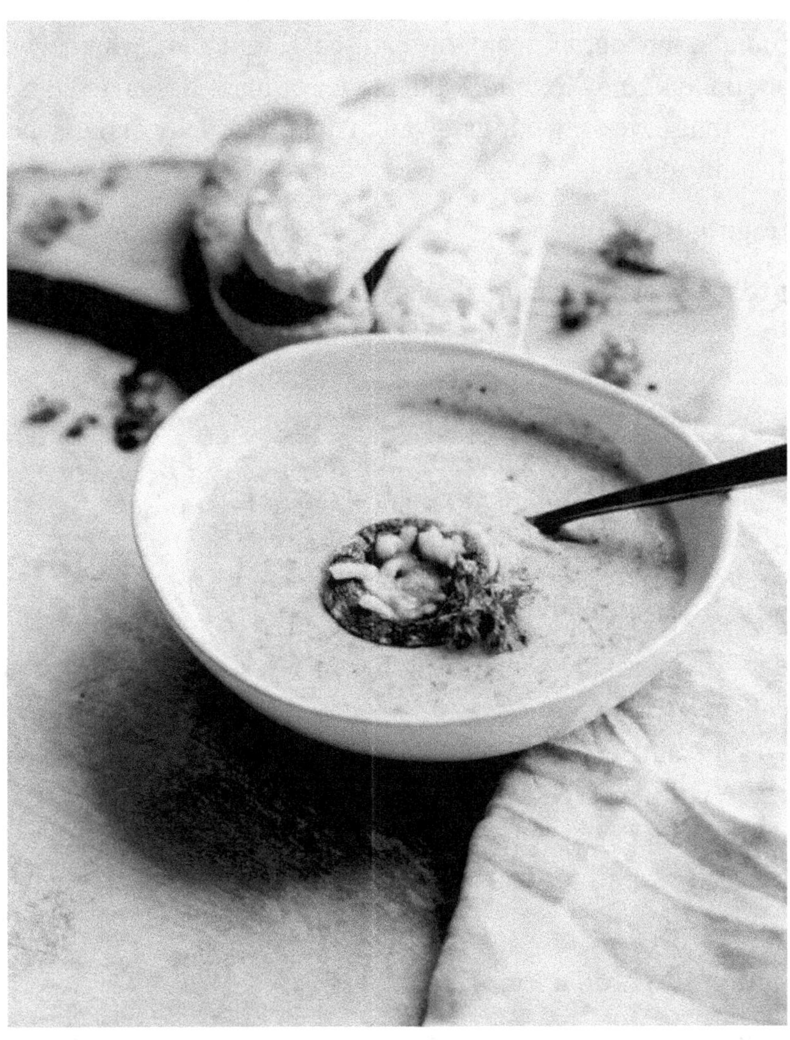

Chapter 2: Vegan & Vegetarian Basics

Welcome to the heart of "Weeknight Vegan & Vegetarian Delights." In this chapter, we'll lay the foundation for your culinary journey into the vibrant and flavorful world of plant-based cooking.

Introduction to Vegan and Vegetarian Cooking: Unlocking the Power of Plant-Based Delights

Welcome to the vibrant realm of plant-based cooking, where we embark on a journey to unlock the power of plant-based delights. This section serves as your gateway to the philosophy and essence of vegan and vegetarian cuisine.

Embracing the Philosophy:

Plant-based cooking is more than a diet; it's a philosophy that revolves around the wholesome goodness of nature. In this exploration, we encourage you to embrace the idea of crafting meals that draw their inspiration from the bounty of fruits, vegetables, grains, and legumes. It's about finding joy in creating dishes that not only nourish your body but also contribute to the well-being of the planet.

Crafting Satisfying and Delicious Meals:

Here, we dive into the art of crafting meals that are both satisfying and delicious, all without relying on animal products. You'll learn how to substitute and enhance flavors, ensuring that every bite is a celebration of the diverse and delicious offerings of the plant kingdom. From hearty stews to vibrant salads, we'll explore a myriad of culinary possibilities that redefine the notion of a satisfying and flavorful meal.

Motivations Behind a Plant-Based Lifestyle:

Understanding the motivations behind choosing a plant-based lifestyle is crucial. Whether you're drawn to this way of eating for health reasons, environmental sustainability, or ethical considerations, we'll explore each aspect. Uncover the wealth of benefits that come with embracing plant-based choices, from improved well-being to contributing to a more sustainable and compassionate world.

Balancing Flavors, Textures, and Nutritional Elements:

Creating delightful plant-based meals is an art that involves balancing flavors, textures, and nutritional elements. This section provides insights into the harmonious combination of ingredients that result in a well-rounded and satisfying dish. From the umami of mushrooms to the crunch of fresh vegetables, you'll learn to orchestrate a symphony of tastes and textures on your plate.

Debunking Myths and Celebrating Creativity:

As we delve deeper, we'll debunk common myths associated with plant-based cooking. Whether it's concerns about protein intake or misconceptions about flavor limitations, we'll address them head-on. Moreover, we celebrate the inherent creativity in plant-based cooking. Far from being restrictive, this culinary approach opens up a world of inventive combinations and flavors, inviting you to explore, experiment, and savor the creativity that lies within every plant-based dish.

In essence, this introduction sets the stage for a fulfilling and flavorful culinary experience. It's an invitation to not just adopt a plant-based diet but to embrace a lifestyle that nourishes both your body and your sense of culinary adventure. Get ready to unlock the delicious potential that plant-based cooking holds!

Essential Ingredients: Building Blocks of Flavor and Nutrition

Welcome to the heart of plant-based creativity—Essential Ingredients. In this section, we embark on a culinary journey through the foundational elements that form the core of plant-based cooking, providing you with the building blocks for both flavor-packed and nutritionally rich meals.

Grains: Quinoa, Farro, and Beyond:

Grains are the sturdy foundation of many plant-based dishes. Quinoa, with its nutty flavor and protein-packed profile, and farro, known for its hearty texture, are just the beginning. We'll explore the diverse world of grains, from brown rice to bulgur, each offering unique textures and nutritional benefits. Uncover the secrets of cooking these grains to perfection, enhancing both taste and nutritional value in your meals.

Legumes: Lentils, Chickpeas, and More:

Legumes add a robust punch to plant-based dishes, bringing in not only protein but also a range of flavors and textures. Lentils, versatile and quick-cooking, join forces with chickpeas, renowned for their creamy texture. Dive into the legume landscape, discovering the potential of black beans, kidney beans, and beyond. Learn how to prepare legumes from scratch and incorporate them into a variety of dishes, from soups to salads, making them a staple in your plant-based pantry.

Colorful Vegetables: Nature's Palette:

Vegetables take center stage in plant-based cooking, offering an array of colors, flavors, and nutrients. From vibrant bell peppers to nutrient-rich leafy greens, we'll explore the diverse world of vegetables and their culinary possibilities. Learn how to maximize the nutritional content of your dishes by incorporating a rainbow of veggies, creating visually appealing and healthful meals that celebrate the freshness of nature.

Plant-Based Proteins: Tofu, Tempeh, and Beyond:

Discover the versatility of plant-based proteins that go beyond the traditional meat substitutes. Tofu, with its chameleon-like ability to absorb flavors, and tempeh, known for its nutty taste and firm texture, open up new dimensions in your plant-based culinary repertoire. We'll guide you through the art of preparing and flavoring these proteins, allowing you to infuse your dishes with a satisfying and protein-rich punch.

Healthy Fats: Avocados, Nuts, and Seeds:

Healthy fats play a crucial role in plant-based cooking, offering not only satiety but also a delightful richness to your meals. Avocados, with their creamy texture, nuts packed with crunch and flavor, and an assortment of seeds providing both texture and nutritional benefits, become your allies in crafting satisfying and well-balanced dishes. Understand the art of incorporating these healthy fats to enhance the overall taste and nutritional profile of your plant-based creations.

Herbs and Spices: Elevating Every Bite:

Herbs and spices are the magic wands in plant-based cooking, transforming ordinary ingredients into extraordinary meals. Explore a palette that includes aromatic basil, earthy cumin, and fiery chili peppers. We'll guide you through the art of seasoning, allowing you to create dishes that are not just nutritious but burst with layers of flavor. Understand the nuances of each herb and spice, empowering you to tailor your meals to suit your taste preferences.

By understanding the role each of these essential ingredients plays, you'll be empowered to create diverse, satisfying, and nourishing plant-based meals. Get ready to turn your kitchen into a vibrant canvas where these ingredients come together to create culinary masterpieces that celebrate the richness of plant-based living!

Cooking Methods: Mastering the Art of Plant-Based Preparation

Welcome to the heart of the kitchen, where the alchemy of plant-based preparation comes to life. In this section, we'll delve into the various cooking methods, unlocking the full potential of plant-based ingredients and guiding you through the art of culinary transformation.

Sautéing: Enhancing Flavors, Preserving Texture:

Sautéing is the quick and dynamic dance of ingredients in a hot pan, a technique that allows you to enhance flavors while preserving the natural textures of vegetables. We'll explore the secrets of the sauté, from choosing the right oils to perfecting the art of achieving that golden caramelization. Whether you're creating a medley of colorful veggies or infusing herbs into your sauté, you'll discover how this method can elevate the taste and texture of your plant-based dishes.

Roasting: Adding Depth and Richness:

Roasting is a slow, patient embrace of ingredients in the oven, a method that adds depth and richness to your plant-based creations. We'll guide you through the nuances of roasting, from selecting the perfect temperature to balancing flavors with herbs and spices. Whether it's hearty root vegetables or the charred perfection of Brussels sprouts, you'll master the technique of roasting, transforming simple ingredients into complex, flavorful delights.

Steaming: Maximum Nutritional Value:

Steaming is the gentle hug of heat that envelops your ingredients, retaining the maximum nutritional value. Dive into the world of steaming, exploring the versatility of this method for vegetables, grains, and even dumplings. Learn the importance of timing and the impact on texture as we guide you through the steps to create dishes that are not only healthful but also bursting with freshness. Steaming becomes your ally in preserving the essence of plant-based goodness.

Stir-Frying: Vibrant and Quick Dishes:

Stir-frying is the energetic waltz of ingredients in a hot wok, a method that creates vibrant and quick plant-based dishes. We'll take you on a journey through the fundamentals of stir-frying, from the right oil for the job to the art of the toss. Whether you're crafting a colorful vegetable stir-fry or experimenting with tofu and tempeh, stir-frying allows you to create meals that are both visually appealing and quick to the table. Discover the secrets to achieving the perfect stir-fry balance, where each ingredient shines.

Guiding You to Optimal Results:

In each method, we're not just providing recipes but guiding you through the principles that lead to optimal results. From the understanding of heat levels to the art of seasoning during and after the cooking process, you'll gain insights into the finer details that make a significant difference in your plant-based dishes. Learn to adapt these methods to different ingredients, allowing you the flexibility to craft a hearty plant-based stew or a refreshing salad with equal finesse.

Whether you're a culinary novice or a seasoned home chef, understanding these cooking techniques will open up a world of possibilities. Get ready to embark on a culinary adventure where each night brings the promise of a delicious and wholesome plant-based meal, crafted with mastery and love.

Chapter 3: Weeknight Dinner Meal Plans

- Week 1

    - Monday: [Recipe]

    - Tuesday: [Recipe]

    - Wednesday: [Recipe]

    - Thursday: [Recipe]

    - Friday: [Recipe]

- Week 2

    - Repeat format for each day

- Week 3

    - Repeat format for each day

- Week 4

    - Repeat format for each day

Chapter 3: Weeknight Dinner Meal Plans

Welcome to a month of delightful weeknight dinner plans designed to simplify your evenings while indulging your taste buds. Each week offers a unique selection of plant-based recipes, ensuring variety, nutrition, and the joy of home-cooked meals for your small family. With serving sizes tailored for 4 to 5 people, these recipes are perfect for enjoying dinner together and having leftovers for a convenient next-day lunch.

Week 1

Monday: Lentil and Vegetable Stew

- A hearty start to the week, this stew combines lentils with a medley of colorful vegetables. Serve over quinoa for a complete and nutritious meal.

Tuesday: Chickpea and Spinach Curry

- Embrace the flavors of India with this quick and flavorful chickpea and spinach curry. Pair it with brown rice for a satisfying dinner.

Wednesday: Mushroom and Thyme Risotto

- Dive into a creamy and comforting mushroom and thyme risotto. This dish is a celebration of rich flavors and tender Arborio rice.

Thursday: Sweet Potato and Black Bean Enchiladas

- Spice up your evening with sweet potato and black bean enchiladas. Topped with a zesty tomato sauce, these enchiladas are a crowd-pleaser.

Friday: Mediterranean Quinoa Salad

- Start your weekend with a light and refreshing Mediterranean quinoa salad. Packed with veggies and olives, it's a perfect way to end the week.

Week 2

Monday: Red Lentil Curry with Cauliflower

- Kick off the week with a protein-packed red lentil curry featuring cauliflower. Serve it over basmati rice for a wholesome and flavorful dinner.

Tuesday: Portobello Mushroom and Polenta Stacks

- Elevate your Tuesday with portobello mushroom and polenta stacks. Layered with marinara sauce and vegan cheese, this dish is a delicious twist on lasagna.

Wednesday: Thai-Inspired Coconut Noodle Soup

- Transport your taste buds to Thailand with a comforting coconut noodle soup. Filled with veggies and aromatic spices, it's a bowl of warmth and flavor.

Thursday: Quinoa-Stuffed Bell Peppers

- Enjoy a colorful and nutritious dinner with quinoa-stuffed bell peppers. Baked to perfection, these peppers are a tasty way to get your veggie fix.

Friday: Black-Eyed Pea and Vegetable Stir-Fry

- Stir-fry your way into the weekend with a vibrant black-eyed pea and vegetable stir-fry. Quick, flavorful, and perfect served over brown rice.

Week 3

Monday: Spinach and Artichoke Stuffed Shells

- Start the week with a classic Italian dish. These spinach and artichoke stuffed shells are baked in marinara sauce for a comforting dinner.

Tuesday: Teriyaki Tofu and Vegetable Skewers

- Add a touch of Asian flair to your Tuesday with teriyaki tofu and vegetable skewers. Grilled to perfection, these skewers are both savory and satisfying.

Wednesday: Mediterranean Chickpea Salad

- Enjoy a light and refreshing Mediterranean chickpea salad. Packed with veggies and tossed in a lemon-herb dressing, it's a perfect midweek dinner.

Thursday: Eggplant and Tomato Bake

- Delight in the simplicity of an eggplant and tomato bake. Layers of roasted vegetables come together in a casserole for a comforting and wholesome meal.

Friday: Spaghetti Aglio e Olio with Roasted Vegetables

- Celebrate the upcoming weekend with a quick and flavorful spaghetti aglio e olio. Roasted vegetables add depth to this classic Italian dish.

Week 4

Monday: Butternut Squash and Sage Risotto

- Begin the last week with a creamy butternut squash and sage risotto. The nutty flavor of the squash and the earthiness of sage create a perfect harmony.

Tuesday: Lentil and Vegetable Curry

- Dive into a spicy lentil and vegetable curry on Tuesday night. Served over basmati rice, it's a satisfying and nutritious meal.

Wednesday: Portobello Mushroom Fajitas

- Spice up your Wednesday with portobello mushroom fajitas. Served with all the classic toppings, these fajitas are a hit with everyone.

Thursday: Quinoa and Black Bean Stuffed Peppers

- Enjoy a different take on stuffed peppers with quinoa and black bean filling. Baked to perfection, these peppers are both wholesome and delicious.

Friday: Mediterranean Chickpea and Spinach Wrap

- Wrap up the week with a quick and satisfying Mediterranean chickpea and spinach wrap. Perfect for a casual and flavorful Friday dinner.

Each week offers a unique culinary journey, ensuring a month filled with delicious, plant-based dinners. Enjoy the convenience of leftovers for lunch the next day and savor the joy of home-cooked meals with your small family. Happy cooking!

Chapter 4: Recipes

- Quick and Easy Dinners

- One-Pot Wonders

- Sheet Pan Delights

- Flavorful Stir-Fries

- Comforting Soups and Stews

- Nutrient-Packed Bowls

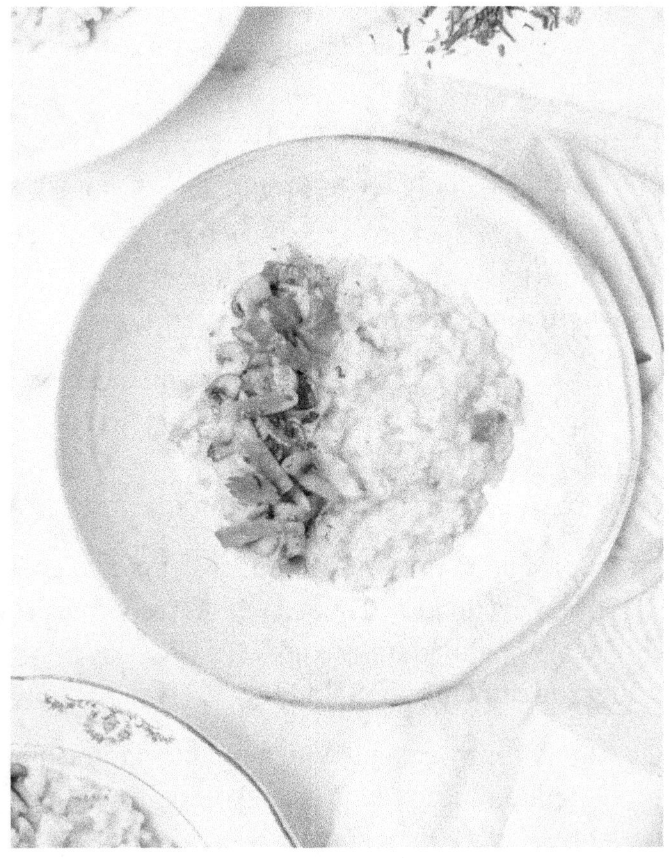

Chapter 4: Recipes

Embark on a culinary journey with a diverse selection of 20 plant-based recipes, carefully organized into six cooking categories to simplify your weeknight dinners. From quick and easy options to comforting soups and stews, each dish promises to bring joy to your table.

Quick and Easy Dinners

1. **Lentil and Vegetable Stew**

   - A hearty stew combining lentils with a medley of colorful vegetables. Serve over quinoa for a complete and nutritious meal.

2. **Chickpea and Spinach Curry**

   - Embrace the flavors of India with this quick and flavorful chickpea and spinach curry. Pair it with brown rice for a satisfying dinner.

3. **Mushroom and Thyme Risotto**

   - Dive into a creamy and comforting mushroom and thyme risotto. This dish is a celebration of rich flavors and tender Arborio rice.

4. **Sweet Potato and Black Bean Enchiladas**

   - Spice up your evening with sweet potato and black bean enchiladas. Topped with a zesty tomato sauce, these enchiladas are a crowd-pleaser.

5. **Mediterranean Quinoa Salad**

   - Start your weekend with a light and refreshing Mediterranean quinoa salad. Packed with veggies and olives, it's a perfect way to end the week.

One-Pot Wonders

6. **Red Lentil Curry with Cauliflower**

- Kick off the week with a protein-packed red lentil curry featuring cauliflower. Serve it over basmati rice for a wholesome and flavorful dinner.

7. **Portobello Mushroom and Polenta Stacks**

- Elevate your Tuesday with portobello mushroom and polenta stacks. Layered with marinara sauce and vegan cheese, this dish is a delicious twist on lasagna.

8. **Thai-Inspired Coconut Noodle Soup**

- Transport your taste buds to Thailand with a comforting coconut noodle soup. Filled with veggies and aromatic spices, it's a bowl of warmth and flavor.

9. **Quinoa-Stuffed Bell Peppers**

- Enjoy a colorful and nutritious dinner with quinoa-stuffed bell peppers. Baked to perfection, these peppers are a tasty way to get your veggie fix.

10. **Black-Eyed Pea and Vegetable Stir-Fry**

- Stir-fry your way into the weekend with a vibrant black-eyed pea and vegetable stir-fry. Quick, flavorful, and perfect served over brown rice.

Sheet Pan Delights

11. **Mediterranean Roasted Vegetable Platter**

- A colorful medley of roasted vegetables, olives, and hummus, served on a sheet pan for a delightful and shareable dinner.

12. **Teriyaki Tofu and Broccoli Sheet Pan**

- Experience the umami of teriyaki-marinated tofu paired with roasted broccoli in this easy and savory sheet pan delight.

Flavorful Stir-Fries

13. **Sesame Ginger Tofu Stir-Fry**

- A sesame ginger-infused stir-fry featuring tofu and an array of colorful vegetables. Quick, flavorful, and perfect over brown rice.

14.   **Pineapple and Cashew Vegetable Stir-Fry**

- Take your taste buds on a tropical journey with this pineapple and cashew vegetable stir-fry, a sweet and savory delight.

15.   **Spicy Peanut Noodle Stir-Fry**

- Kick up the heat with a spicy peanut noodle stir-fry, combining udon noodles with a medley of veggies for a satisfying dish.

Comforting Soups and Stews

16.   **Butternut Squash and Lentil Soup**

- Cozy up with a bowl of butternut squash and lentil soup, flavored with warming spices for a comforting and nourishing experience.

17.   **Minestrone with White Beans and Kale**

- A hearty minestrone soup filled with white beans, kale, and a medley of vegetables. Satisfying and perfect for chilly evenings.

18.   **Red Curry Chickpea and Vegetable Stew**

- Embrace the bold flavors of red curry in this chickpea and vegetable stew, a hearty and aromatic option for a satisfying dinner.

Nutrient-Packed Bowls

19.   **Mushroom and Thyme Risotto**

- Dive into a creamy and comforting mushroom and thyme risotto. This dish is a celebration of rich flavors and tender Arborio rice.

20.   **Spinach and Artichoke Stuffed Shells**

- Start the week with a classic Italian dish. These spinach and artichoke stuffed shells are baked in marinara sauce for a comforting dinner.

Savor the simplicity and deliciousness of these recipes, perfect for a small family. Incorporating the weeknight dinner meal plans from Chapter 3, these dishes offer variety and nutrition, ensuring your weeknight dinners are both enjoyable and convenient. Happy cooking!

Quick and Easy Dinners

Lentil and Vegetable Stew

Ingredients:

- 1 cup dried green lentils
- 2 cups vegetable broth
- 1 onion, diced
- 2 carrots, sliced
- 2 celery stalks, chopped
- 3 cloves garlic, minced
- 1 can (14 oz) diced tomatoes
- 1 teaspoon cumin
- 1 teaspoon paprika
- Salt and pepper to taste
- 4 cups cooked quinoa (for serving)

Nutrition Benefits:

- High in plant-based protein and fiber from lentils.
- Abundance of vitamins and minerals from vegetables.

Total Time:

- Preparation: 15 minutes
- Cooking: 30 minutes
- Total: 45 minutes

Instructions:

1. In a large pot, sauté the diced onion, carrots, and celery until softened.
2. Add the minced garlic and cook for an additional 1-2 minutes until fragrant.
3. Pour in the vegetable broth, diced tomatoes, lentils, cumin, paprika, salt, and pepper. Bring to a boil.
4. Reduce heat to a simmer, cover, and let it cook for about 25-30 minutes or until lentils are tender.

5. Serve the stew over cooked quinoa. Enjoy the hearty goodness!

Chickpea and Spinach Curry

Ingredients:

- 2 cans (15 oz each) chickpeas, drained and rinsed
- 1 onion, finely chopped
- 3 tomatoes, diced
- 2 cups spinach, washed and chopped
- 1 can (14 oz) coconut milk
- 3 tablespoons curry powder
- 1 teaspoon turmeric
- Salt to taste
- Cooked brown rice (for serving)

Nutrition Benefits:

- Rich in plant-based protein and iron from chickpeas.
- Abundant in vitamins and minerals from spinach and tomatoes.

Total Time:

- Preparation: 20 minutes
- Cooking: 25 minutes
- Total: 45 minutes

Instructions:

1. In a large pan, sauté the chopped onion until golden brown.
2. Add the diced tomatoes, curry powder, turmeric, and salt. Cook until tomatoes are soft.
3. Pour in the coconut milk and bring the mixture to a simmer.
4. Add the chickpeas and spinach. Simmer for an additional 10-15 minutes until the spinach wilts.
5. Serve the curry over cooked brown rice. Enjoy the aromatic flavors!

Mushroom and Thyme Risotto

Ingredients:

- 2 cups Arborio rice
- 1 pound mushrooms (button or cremini), sliced
- 1 onion, finely chopped
- 4 cloves garlic, minced
- 1 cup dry white wine
- 6 cups vegetable broth, kept warm
- 2 tablespoons fresh thyme leaves
- 1/2 cup nutritional yeast (optional, for a cheesy flavor)
- Salt and black pepper to taste

Nutrition Benefits:

- Good source of complex carbohydrates from Arborio rice.
- Mushrooms provide essential nutrients like vitamin D.

Total Time:

- Preparation: 15 minutes
- Cooking: 25 minutes
- Total: 40 minutes

Instructions:

1. In a large pan, sauté the chopped onion and garlic until softened.
2. Add the sliced mushrooms and cook until they release their moisture.
3. Stir in the Arborio rice and cook for 2-3 minutes until lightly toasted.
4. Pour in the white wine and cook until it's mostly absorbed.
5. Begin adding the warm vegetable broth, one ladle at a time, stirring frequently until the liquid is absorbed before adding more.
6. Continue this process until the rice is creamy and cooked to al dente.

7. Stir in thyme leaves, nutritional yeast (if using), salt, and black pepper.
8. Serve the risotto hot. Enjoy the creamy and savory goodness!

Sweet Potato and Black Bean Enchiladas

Ingredients:

- 2 medium sweet potatoes, peeled and diced
- 1 can (15 oz) black beans, drained and rinsed
- 1 red onion, finely chopped
- 1 teaspoon cumin
- 1 teaspoon chili powder
- 1/2 teaspoon smoked paprika
- 8 small whole wheat tortillas
- 1 can (14 oz) enchilada sauce
- 1 cup vegan cheese, shredded
- Fresh cilantro, chopped (for garnish)

Nutrition Benefits:

- Sweet potatoes offer vitamins and fiber.
- Black beans contribute plant-based protein and fiber.

Total Time:

- Preparation: 20 minutes
- Cooking: 25 minutes
- Total: 45 minutes

Instructions:

1. Steam or boil the diced sweet potatoes until tender. Mash them in a bowl.
2. In a pan, sauté the chopped red onion until translucent.
3. Add the black beans, cumin, chili powder, and smoked paprika. Cook for an additional 5 minutes.
4. Warm the tortillas and fill each with a spoonful of mashed sweet potatoes and the black bean mixture.

5. Roll the tortillas and place them seam-side down in a baking dish.
6. Pour the enchilada sauce over the top and sprinkle with vegan cheese.
7. Bake in the oven at 375°F (190°C) for 20 minutes or until the cheese is melted and bubbly.
8. Garnish with fresh cilantro and serve. Enjoy the delicious and spicy kick!

Mediterranean Quinoa Salad

Ingredients:

- 2 cups cooked quinoa
- 1 cucumber, diced
- 1 cup cherry tomatoes, halved
- 1/2 red onion, finely chopped
- 1/2 cup Kalamata olives, pitted and sliced
- 1/2 cup fresh parsley, chopped
- 1/4 cup extra-virgin olive oil
- 2 tablespoons red wine vinegar
- Salt and black pepper to taste

Nutrition Benefits:

- Quinoa provides a complete protein source.
- Cucumbers and tomatoes offer vitamins and hydration.

Total Time:

- Preparation: 15 minutes
- Cooking: 15 minutes (for quinoa)
- Total: 30 minutes

Instructions:

1. In a large bowl, combine the cooked quinoa, diced cucumber, cherry tomatoes, chopped red onion, olives, and fresh parsley.
2. In a small bowl, whisk together the olive oil, red wine vinegar, salt, and black pepper to create the dressing.

3. Pour the dressing over the quinoa mixture and toss until well combined.
4. Refrigerate for at least 15 minutes to let the flavors meld.
5. Serve the Mediterranean quinoa salad chilled. Enjoy the refreshing and nutrient-packed dish!

One-Pot Wonders

Red Lentil Curry with Cauliflower

Ingredients:

- 1 cup red lentils, rinsed and drained
- 1 cauliflower, cut into florets
- 1 onion, finely chopped
- 3 cloves garlic, minced
- 1 can (14 oz) coconut milk
- 1 can (14 oz) diced tomatoes
- 2 tablespoons red curry paste
- 1 teaspoon ground turmeric
- 1 teaspoon ground cumin
- Salt and black pepper to taste
- Fresh cilantro, chopped (for garnish)
- Cooked basmati rice (for serving)

Nutrition Benefits:

- Red lentils provide protein and fiber.
- Cauliflower adds vitamins and minerals.

Total Time:

- Preparation: 15 minutes
- Cooking: 25 minutes
- Total: 40 minutes

Instructions:

1. In a large pot, combine red lentils, cauliflower florets, chopped onion, minced garlic, coconut milk, diced tomatoes, red curry paste, ground turmeric, ground cumin, salt, and black pepper.
2. Bring the mixture to a boil, then reduce heat to a simmer. Cook for about 20-25 minutes or until lentils are tender.
3. Stir occasionally to prevent sticking. Adjust seasoning if necessary.

4. Serve the red lentil curry over cooked basmati rice.
5. Garnish with fresh cilantro. Enjoy this protein-packed curry with the goodness of cauliflower!

Portobello Mushroom and Polenta Stacks

Ingredients:

- 4 portobello mushrooms, stems removed
- 1 cup polenta, sliced into rounds
- 2 cups marinara sauce
- 1 cup vegan mozzarella cheese, shredded
- Fresh basil leaves (for garnish)

Nutrition Benefits:

- Portobello mushrooms provide a meaty texture.
- Polenta offers a comforting and filling base.

Total Time:

- Preparation: 15 minutes
- Cooking: 25 minutes
- Total: 40 minutes

Instructions:

1. Preheat the oven to 375°F (190°C).
2. In a baking dish, layer portobello mushrooms with polenta rounds, marinara sauce, and vegan mozzarella cheese.
3. Repeat the layers until ingredients are used, finishing with a layer of marinara sauce and cheese on top.
4. Bake for 20-25 minutes or until the cheese is melted and bubbly.
5. Remove from the oven, garnish with fresh basil leaves, and let it cool slightly before serving.
6. Enjoy these delicious portobello mushroom and polenta stacks, a delightful twist on traditional lasagna!

Thai-Inspired Coconut Noodle Soup

Ingredients:

- 8 oz rice noodles
- 1 can (14 oz) coconut milk
- 4 cups vegetable broth
- 1 cup broccoli florets
- 1 carrot, julienned
- 1 red bell pepper, sliced
- 1 cup tofu, cubed
- 2 tablespoons soy sauce
- 1 tablespoon red curry paste
- 1 tablespoon lime juice
- Fresh cilantro and lime wedges (for garnish)

Nutrition Benefits:

- Rice noodles provide a gluten-free option.
- Coconut milk adds richness to the soup.

Total Time:

- Preparation: 15 minutes
- Cooking: 20 minutes
- Total: 35 minutes

Instructions:

1. Cook rice noodles according to package instructions. Drain and set aside.
2. In a large pot, combine coconut milk, vegetable broth, broccoli florets, julienned carrot, sliced red bell pepper, cubed tofu, soy sauce, red curry paste, and lime juice.
3. Bring the mixture to a simmer and cook for about 15-20 minutes until vegetables are tender.
4. Adjust seasoning if necessary.
5. Divide the cooked rice noodles into serving bowls and ladle the hot soup over them.

6. Garnish with fresh cilantro and lime wedges. Enjoy the comforting warmth of this Thai-inspired coconut noodle soup!

Quinoa-Stuffed Bell Peppers

Ingredients:

- 1 cup quinoa, cooked
- 4 bell peppers, halved and seeds removed
- 1 can (14 oz) black beans, drained and rinsed
- 1 cup corn kernels (fresh or frozen)
- 1 cup cherry tomatoes, halved
- 1 teaspoon ground cumin
- 1 teaspoon chili powder
- Salt and black pepper to taste
- 1 cup vegan shredded cheese
- Fresh cilantro, chopped (for garnish)

Nutrition Benefits:

- Quinoa offers a complete protein source.
- Bell peppers provide vitamins and antioxidants.

Total Time:

- Preparation: 20 minutes
- Cooking: 25 minutes
- Total: 45 minutes

Instructions:

1. Preheat the oven to 375°F (190°C).
2. In a bowl, combine cooked quinoa, black beans, corn, cherry tomatoes, ground cumin, chili powder, salt, and black pepper.
3. Stuff the halved bell peppers with the quinoa mixture and place them in a baking dish.
4. Top each stuffed pepper with vegan shredded cheese.
5. Bake for 20-25 minutes or until the peppers are tender and the cheese is melted.

6. Garnish with fresh cilantro and serve. Enjoy these colorful and nutritious quinoa-stuffed bell peppers!

Black-Eyed Pea and Vegetable Stir-Fry

Ingredients:

- 2 cups black-eyed peas, cooked
- 2 cups broccoli florets
- 1 red bell pepper, sliced
- 1 yellow bell pepper, sliced
- 1 carrot, julienned
- 1 cup snap peas, trimmed
- 3 tablespoons soy sauce
- 1 tablespoon sesame oil
- 1 teaspoon ginger, minced
- 2 cloves garlic, minced
- 1 tablespoon sesame seeds (for garnish)
- Cooked brown rice (for serving)

Nutrition Benefits:

- Black-eyed peas offer plant-based protein and fiber.
- Colorful vegetables provide a variety of vitamins and minerals.

Total Time:

- Preparation: 15 minutes
- Cooking: 15 minutes
- Total: 30 minutes

Instructions:

1. In a wok or large skillet, heat sesame oil over medium-high heat. Add minced ginger and garlic, and sauté for 1-2 minutes.
2. Add broccoli, red bell pepper, yellow bell pepper, julienned carrot, and snap peas to the wok. Stir-fry for about 5-7 minutes until the vegetables are crisp-tender.

3. Add cooked black-eyed peas and soy sauce to the wok. Stir-fry for an additional 3-5 minutes to heat through.
4. Adjust seasoning if necessary.
5. Serve the black-eyed pea and vegetable stir-fry over cooked brown rice.
6. Garnish with sesame seeds and enjoy this vibrant and flavorful stir-fry!

Note: Total time includes both preparation and cooking times.

Sheet Pan Delights

Mediterranean Roasted Vegetable Platter

Ingredients:

- 1 eggplant, sliced
- 1 zucchini, sliced
- 1 red bell pepper, sliced
- 1 yellow bell pepper, sliced
- 1 cup cherry tomatoes
- 1 red onion, thinly sliced
- 1/4 cup Kalamata olives, pitted
- 2 tablespoons olive oil
- 1 teaspoon dried oregano
- 1 teaspoon dried thyme
- Salt and black pepper to taste
- Hummus (for serving)
- Fresh parsley, chopped (for garnish)

Nutrition Benefits:

- Colorful vegetables provide a range of vitamins and antioxidants.
- Olive oil adds heart-healthy monounsaturated fats.

Total Time:

- Preparation: 15 minutes
- Cooking: 25 minutes
- Total: 40 minutes

Instructions:

1. Preheat the oven to 400°F (200°C).
2. In a large bowl, toss sliced eggplant, zucchini, red bell pepper, yellow bell pepper, cherry tomatoes, red onion, olives, olive oil, dried oregano, dried thyme, salt, and black pepper until well-coated.
3. Spread the mixture evenly on a sheet pan.

4. Roast in the preheated oven for 20-25 minutes or until the vegetables are tender and slightly caramelized.
5. Serve the roasted vegetables on a platter, accompanied by hummus.
6. Garnish with fresh parsley. Enjoy this Mediterranean-inspired roasted vegetable platter as a colorful and shareable dinner!

Teriyaki Tofu and Broccoli Sheet Pan

Ingredients:

- 1 block firm tofu, pressed and cubed
- 3 cups broccoli florets
- 1 red bell pepper, sliced
- 1 yellow bell pepper, sliced
- 1/4 cup teriyaki sauce
- 2 tablespoons soy sauce
- 1 tablespoon sesame oil
- 1 tablespoon maple syrup
- 1 teaspoon garlic powder
- 1 teaspoon ginger, minced
- Sesame seeds (for garnish)
- Green onions, sliced (for garnish)
- Cooked brown rice (for serving)

Nutrition Benefits:

- Tofu provides plant-based protein.
- Broccoli is rich in fiber and antioxidants.

Total Time:

- Preparation: 15 minutes
- Cooking: 25 minutes
- Total: 40 minutes

Instructions:

1. Preheat the oven to 400°F (200°C).

2. In a bowl, combine cubed tofu, broccoli florets, sliced red bell pepper, sliced yellow bell pepper, teriyaki sauce, soy sauce, sesame oil, maple syrup, garlic powder, and minced ginger. Toss until tofu and vegetables are evenly coated.
3. Spread the mixture on a sheet pan.
4. Roast in the preheated oven for 20-25 minutes or until the tofu is golden and the broccoli is tender.
5. Remove from the oven and sprinkle with sesame seeds and sliced green onions.
6. Serve the teriyaki tofu and broccoli over cooked brown rice. Enjoy this easy and savory sheet pan delight!

Note: Total time includes both preparation and cooking times.

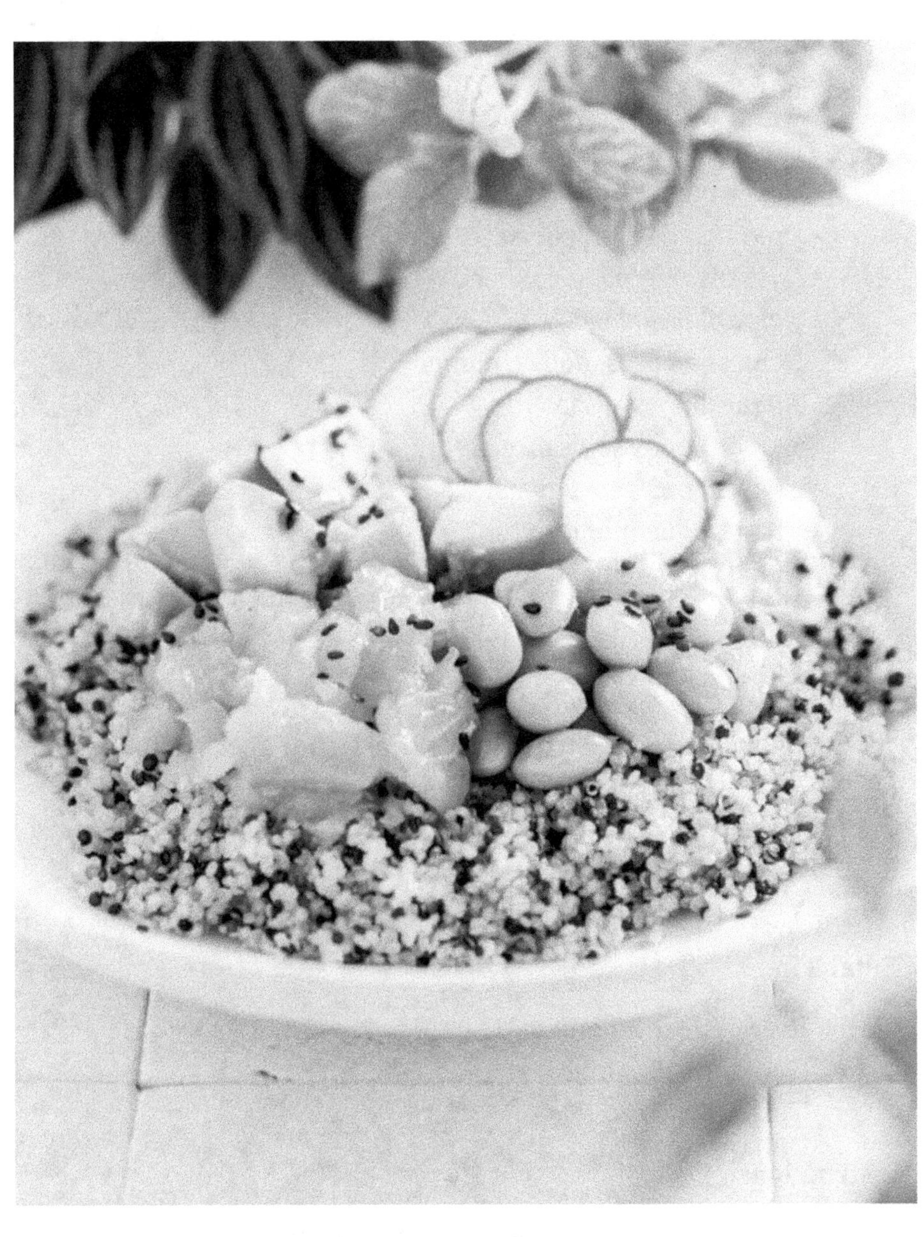

Flavorful Stir-Fries

Sesame Ginger Tofu Stir-Fry

Ingredients:

- 1 block firm tofu, pressed and cubed
- 2 cups broccoli florets
- 1 red bell pepper, sliced
- 1 yellow bell pepper, sliced
- 1 carrot, julienned
- 1 cup snap peas, ends trimmed
- 2 tablespoons sesame oil
- 3 tablespoons soy sauce
- 1 tablespoon rice vinegar
- 1 tablespoon maple syrup
- 1 tablespoon ginger, minced
- 2 cloves garlic, minced
- 1 tablespoon sesame seeds (for garnish)
- Green onions, sliced (for garnish)
- Cooked brown rice (for serving)

Nutrition Benefits:

- Tofu provides plant-based protein.
- Vegetables offer a variety of vitamins and minerals.

Total Time:

- Preparation: 20 minutes
- Cooking: 15 minutes
- Total: 35 minutes

Instructions:

1. In a wok or large skillet, heat sesame oil over medium-high heat.

2. Add cubed tofu and stir-fry until golden brown on all sides. Remove tofu from the wok and set aside.
3. In the same wok, add more sesame oil if needed. Stir-fry broccoli, red bell pepper, yellow bell pepper, carrot, and snap peas until vegetables are tender-crisp.
4. In a small bowl, whisk together soy sauce, rice vinegar, maple syrup, minced ginger, and minced garlic.
5. Add the cooked tofu back to the wok and pour the sauce over the tofu and vegetables. Toss to coat evenly.
6. Continue cooking for 2-3 minutes until everything is heated through.
7. Serve the sesame ginger tofu stir-fry over cooked brown rice, garnished with sesame seeds and sliced green onions.

Pineapple and Cashew Vegetable Stir-Fry

Ingredients:

- 1 cup pineapple chunks (fresh or canned)
- 1 cup broccoli florets
- 1 red bell pepper, sliced
- 1 yellow bell pepper, sliced
- 1 cup snow peas, ends trimmed
- 1/2 cup cashews, toasted
- 2 tablespoons soy sauce
- 1 tablespoon hoisin sauce
- 1 tablespoon rice vinegar
- 1 tablespoon maple syrup
- 1 tablespoon vegetable oil
- 1 teaspoon ginger, minced
- 2 cloves garlic, minced
- Cooked jasmine rice (for serving)

Nutrition Benefits:

- Pineapple adds natural sweetness and vitamin C.
- Cashews contribute healthy fats and protein.

Total Time:

- Preparation: 15 minutes
- Cooking: 10 minutes
- Total: 25 minutes

Instructions:

1. In a wok or large skillet, heat vegetable oil over medium-high heat.
2. Stir-fry broccoli, red bell pepper, yellow bell pepper, and snow peas until vegetables are slightly tender.
3. Add pineapple chunks and toasted cashews to the wok.
4. In a small bowl, whisk together soy sauce, hoisin sauce, rice vinegar, maple syrup, minced ginger, and minced garlic.
5. Pour the sauce over the stir-fry and toss to coat evenly.
6. Continue cooking for an additional 2-3 minutes until everything is heated through.
7. Serve the pineapple and cashew vegetable stir-fry over cooked jasmine rice.

Spicy Peanut Noodle Stir-Fry

Ingredients:

- 8 oz udon noodles, cooked according to package instructions
- 1 cup broccoli florets
- 1 red bell pepper, sliced
- 1 yellow bell pepper, sliced
- 1 cup shredded cabbage
- 1/2 cup shredded carrots
- 1/3 cup peanuts, chopped
- 3 tablespoons soy sauce
- 2 tablespoons peanut butter
- 1 tablespoon sriracha sauce
- 1 tablespoon rice vinegar
- 1 tablespoon sesame oil
- 1 tablespoon maple syrup

- 2 cloves garlic, minced
- Green onions, sliced (for garnish)

Nutrition Benefits:

- Udon noodles provide a source of complex carbohydrates.
- Peanuts offer healthy fats and protein.

Total Time:

- Preparation: 15 minutes
- Cooking: 10 minutes
- Total: 25 minutes

Instructions:

1. In a wok or large skillet, whisk together soy sauce, peanut butter, sriracha sauce, rice vinegar, sesame oil, maple syrup, and minced garlic over medium heat.
2. Add cooked udon noodles to the wok and toss to coat in the sauce.
3. Stir-fry broccoli, red bell pepper, yellow bell pepper, shredded cabbage, and shredded carrots until vegetables are tender.
4. Add chopped peanuts to the wok and toss to combine.
5. Continue cooking for an additional 2-3 minutes until everything is heated through.
6. Serve the spicy peanut noodle stir-fry, garnished with sliced green onions.

Note: Total time includes both preparation and cooking times.

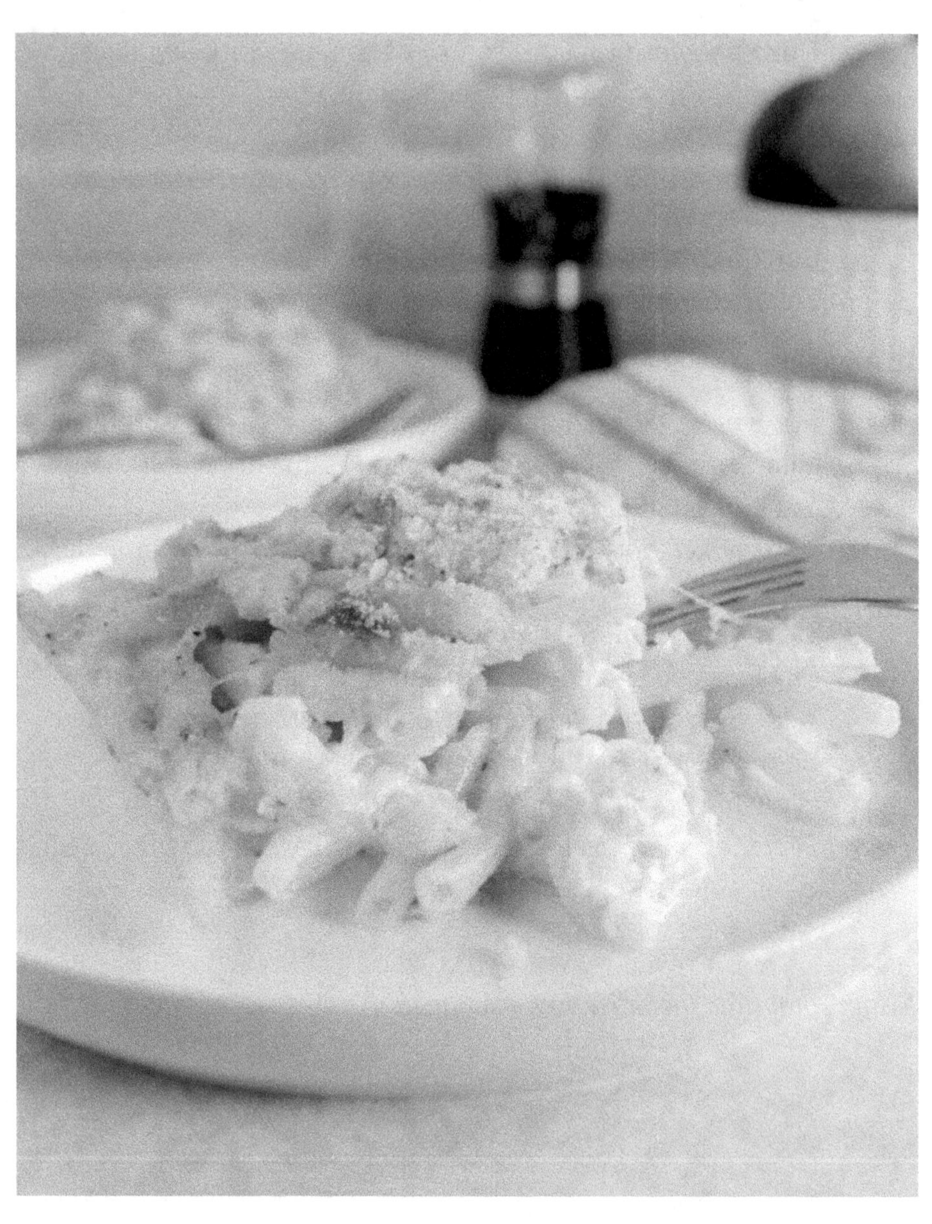

Comforting Soups and Stews

Butternut Squash and Lentil Soup

Ingredients:

- 1 medium butternut squash, peeled and diced
- 1 cup dried brown lentils, rinsed
- 1 onion, diced
- 2 carrots, sliced
- 2 celery stalks, chopped
- 3 cloves garlic, minced
- 1 teaspoon ground cumin
- 1 teaspoon ground coriander
- 1/2 teaspoon smoked paprika
- 1/4 teaspoon cayenne pepper (optional for heat)
- 6 cups vegetable broth
- Salt and black pepper to taste
- 2 tablespoons olive oil
- Fresh parsley, chopped (for garnish)
- Crusty bread (for serving)

Nutrition Benefits:

- Butternut squash provides vitamins A and C.
- Lentils offer plant-based protein and fiber.

Total Time:

- Preparation: 20 minutes
- Cooking: 30 minutes
- Total: 50 minutes

Instructions:

1. In a large pot, heat olive oil over medium heat. Add diced onion, carrots, and celery. Sauté until vegetables are softened.
2. Add minced garlic, ground cumin, ground coriander, smoked paprika, and cayenne pepper (if using). Stir and cook for an additional 2 minutes.

3. Add diced butternut squash, dried brown lentils, and vegetable broth to the pot. Season with salt and black pepper.
4. Bring the soup to a boil, then reduce the heat and simmer for 25-30 minutes or until the lentils and butternut squash are tender.
5. Use an immersion blender to partially blend the soup for a creamy texture while leaving some chunks for texture.
6. Adjust the seasoning if needed. Serve the butternut squash and lentil soup hot, garnished with fresh parsley. Enjoy with crusty bread.

Minestrone with White Beans and Kale

Ingredients:

- 1 can (15 oz) white beans, drained and rinsed
- 1 bunch kale, stems removed and leaves torn into bite-sized pieces
- 1 onion, diced
- 2 carrots, sliced
- 2 celery stalks, chopped
- 3 cloves garlic, minced
- 1 can (28 oz) diced tomatoes
- 6 cups vegetable broth
- 1 teaspoon dried oregano
- 1 teaspoon dried basil
- 1/2 teaspoon dried thyme
- Salt and black pepper to taste
- 2 tablespoons olive oil
- Grated Parmesan cheese (for garnish)
- Crusty bread (for serving)

Nutrition Benefits:

- Kale is rich in vitamins K, A, and C.
- White beans provide protein and fiber.

Total Time:

- Preparation: 15 minutes
- Cooking: 25 minutes
- Total: 40 minutes

Instructions:

1. In a large pot, heat olive oil over medium heat. Add diced onion, carrots, and celery. Sauté until vegetables are softened.
2. Add minced garlic, dried oregano, dried basil, and dried thyme. Stir and cook for an additional 2 minutes.
3. Pour in diced tomatoes and vegetable broth. Season with salt and black pepper.
4. Bring the soup to a boil, then reduce the heat and simmer for 15 minutes.
5. Add white beans and torn kale to the pot. Simmer for an additional 5-7 minutes until the kale is wilted.
6. Adjust the seasoning if needed. Serve the minestrone with white beans and kale hot, garnished with grated Parmesan cheese. Enjoy with crusty bread.

Red Curry Chickpea and Vegetable Stew

Ingredients:

- 2 cans (15 oz each) chickpeas, drained and rinsed
- 1 eggplant, diced
- 1 red bell pepper, sliced
- 1 yellow bell pepper, sliced
- 1 zucchini, sliced
- 1 can (14 oz) coconut milk
- 2 tablespoons red curry paste
- 1 tablespoon soy sauce
- 1 tablespoon maple syrup
- 1 tablespoon vegetable oil
- 2 teaspoons ginger, minced
- 2 cloves garlic, minced
- Fresh cilantro, chopped (for garnish)

- Cooked jasmine rice (for serving)

Nutrition Benefits:

- Chickpeas offer protein and fiber.
- Vegetables provide a variety of vitamins and minerals.

Total Time:

- Preparation: 20 minutes
- Cooking: 25 minutes
- Total: 45 minutes

Instructions:

1. In a large pot, heat vegetable oil over medium heat. Add diced eggplant, sliced red bell pepper, sliced yellow bell pepper, and sliced zucchini. Sauté until vegetables are slightly softened.
2. Add minced ginger and minced garlic to the pot. Stir and cook for an additional 2 minutes.
3. Pour in coconut milk, red curry paste, soy sauce, and maple syrup. Stir until well combined.
4. Add chickpeas to the pot and simmer for 15-20 minutes until the vegetables are tender.
5. Adjust the seasoning if needed. Serve the red curry chickpea and vegetable stew hot, garnished with fresh cilantro. Enjoy over cooked jasmine rice.

Note: Total time includes both preparation and cooking times.

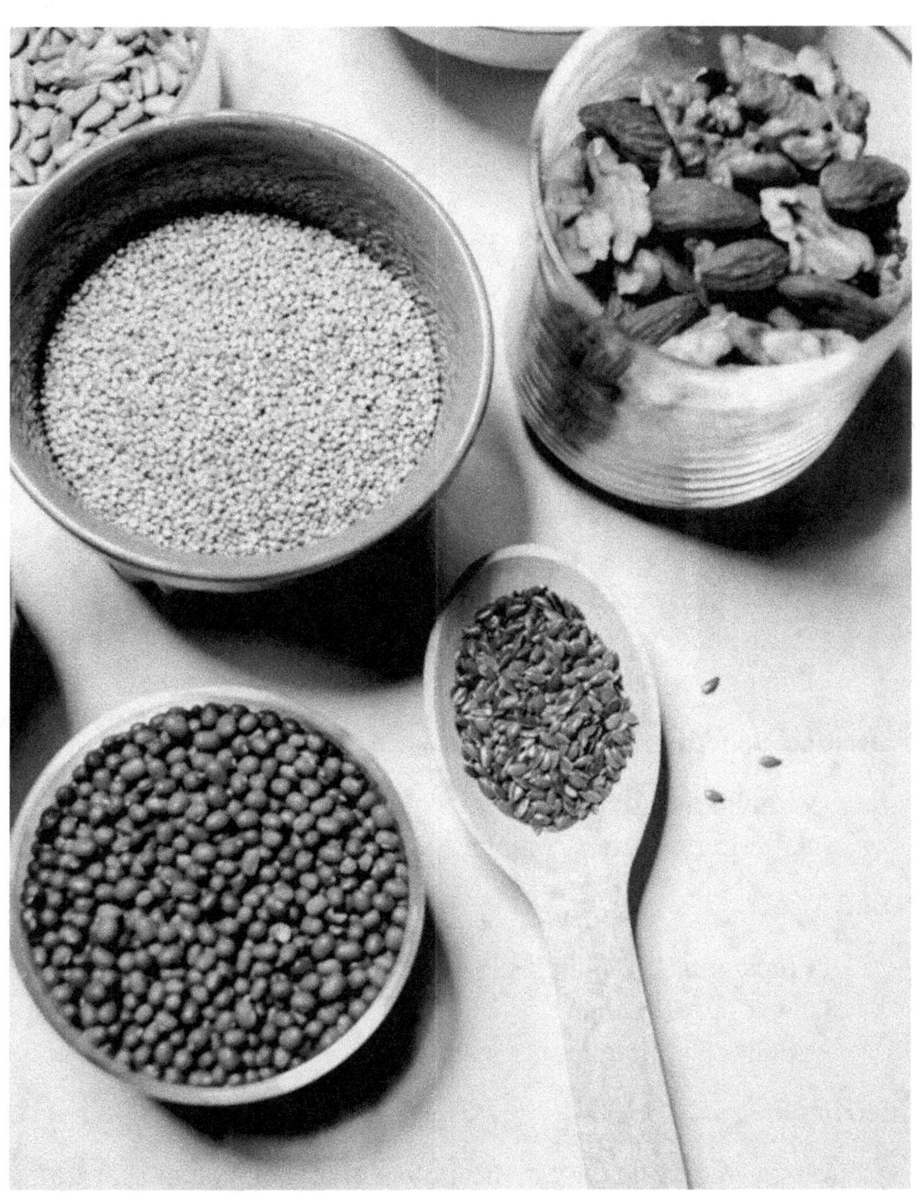

Nutrient-Packed Bowls

Mushroom and Thyme Risotto Bowl

Ingredients:

- 2 cups Arborio rice
- 1 pound cremini mushrooms, sliced
- 1 onion, finely chopped
- 3 cloves garlic, minced
- 4 cups vegetable broth, warmed
- 1 cup dry white wine
- 1 teaspoon fresh thyme leaves
- 1/2 cup nutritional yeast (optional, for a cheesy flavor)
- Salt and black pepper to taste
- 2 tablespoons olive oil
- Fresh parsley, chopped (for garnish)
- Lemon wedges (for serving)

Nutrition Benefits:

- Cremini mushrooms provide vitamins and minerals.
- Arborio rice offers complex carbohydrates.

Total Time:

- Preparation: 15 minutes
- Cooking: 30 minutes
- Total: 45 minutes

Instructions:

1. In a large skillet or pan, heat olive oil over medium heat. Add chopped onion and sauté until translucent.
2. Add sliced cremini mushrooms to the pan and cook until they release their moisture and become golden brown.
3. Stir in minced garlic and Arborio rice. Toast the rice for 2-3 minutes until it becomes lightly golden.
4. Pour in dry white wine and cook until it's mostly absorbed by the rice.

5. Begin adding warm vegetable broth, one ladle at a time, stirring frequently. Allow the liquid to be absorbed before adding the next ladle.
6. Continue this process until the Arborio rice is creamy and cooked to al dente texture.
7. Stir in fresh thyme leaves, nutritional yeast (if using), salt, and black pepper. Adjust the seasoning to taste.
8. Serve the mushroom and thyme risotto in bowls, garnished with fresh parsley. Squeeze lemon wedges over the risotto for a burst of citrus flavor.

Spinach and Artichoke Stuffed Shells Bowl

Ingredients:

- 1 box jumbo pasta shells, cooked according to package instructions
- 2 cups baby spinach, chopped
- 1 can (14 oz) artichoke hearts, drained and chopped
- 1 cup vegan ricotta cheese
- 1/2 cup nutritional yeast
- 2 cloves garlic, minced
- 1 teaspoon dried oregano
- 1 teaspoon dried basil
- Salt and black pepper to taste
- 2 cups marinara sauce
- Vegan mozzarella cheese, shredded (for topping)
- Fresh basil, chopped (for garnish)

Nutrition Benefits:

- Spinach is rich in iron and vitamins.
- Artichoke hearts provide dietary fiber and antioxidants.

Total Time:

- Preparation: 20 minutes
- Cooking: 25 minutes
- Total: 45 minutes

Instructions:

1. Preheat the oven to 375°F (190°C).
2. In a mixing bowl, combine chopped baby spinach, chopped artichoke hearts, vegan ricotta cheese, nutritional yeast, minced garlic, dried oregano, dried basil, salt, and black pepper.
3. Stuff each cooked jumbo pasta shell with the spinach and artichoke mixture.
4. Spread a thin layer of marinara sauce on the bottom of a baking dish.
5. Arrange the stuffed shells in the baking dish and cover them with the remaining marinara sauce.
6. Sprinkle shredded vegan mozzarella cheese over the top.
7. Bake in the preheated oven for 20-25 minutes or until the cheese is melted and bubbly.
8. Garnish with fresh basil before serving the spinach and artichoke stuffed shells bowl.

Note: Total time includes both preparation and cooking times.

Chapter 5: Leftover Lunch Ideas

Creative Ways to Repurpose Dinner Leftovers

Unlock the potential of last night's dinner with these creative and simple ways to transform leftovers into exciting lunches. Repurposing leftovers not only minimizes food waste but also adds a touch of variety to your midday meals. Let's explore some innovative ideas to give your dinner remnants a delicious makeover.

1. Remixing Salads:

Take leftover roasted vegetables, grains, or proteins and toss them into a bed of fresh greens. Drizzle with a new dressing or add some crunchy toppings like nuts or seeds to create a refreshing and satisfying salad.

2. Wrap and Roll:

Transform last night's stir-fry or roasted vegetables into a flavorful wrap or roll. Use whole-grain tortillas or wraps, add a spread like hummus or avocado, and roll up your leftovers for a convenient and portable lunch.

3. Soup Up Leftovers:

Turn stews, curries, or grain-based dishes into a hearty soup by adding some vegetable or broth base. Let it simmer for a few minutes, and you'll have a comforting and warm lunch option.

4. Pizza Redux:

Reimagine leftover saucy dishes as a pizza topping. Spread tomato sauce on a flatbread or tortilla, add your leftovers, sprinkle with vegan cheese, and bake for a quick and tasty pizza lunch.

5. Pasta Salad Transformation:

Give new life to leftover pasta dishes by turning them into a cold pasta salad. Add fresh veggies, a zesty vinaigrette, and perhaps some extra protein like beans or tofu for a delightful pasta salad.

6. Grain Bowl Remix:

Create a customizable grain bowl by combining leftover grains, proteins, and vegetables. Top it with your favorite sauce or dressing and add some greens for a wholesome and filling lunch.

7. Frittata Fusion:

Repurpose roasted or sautéed vegetables into a delicious frittata. Beat some eggs, pour them over the vegetables in a pan, and bake for a protein-packed lunch option.

Lunchbox-Friendly Recipes

For those busy days when you need a lunch that travels well, these lunchbox-friendly recipes are here to save the day. Packed with flavor, nutrition, and easy portability, these recipes ensure you enjoy a satisfying midday meal wherever your day takes you.

1. Quinoa Salad Jars:

Layer cooked quinoa, roasted vegetables, and a flavorful dressing in a jar for a convenient and colorful lunch. Shake it up before eating, and you have a fresh and crisp quinoa salad.

2. Veggie Wrap Packs:

Wrap up your favorite vegetables, hummus, and some leftover protein in a whole-grain wrap. Slice it into bite-sized pinwheels for a delightful and mess-free lunchbox option.

3. Bento Box Delights:

Create a bento box with compartments for a variety of leftovers. Include a mix of grains, proteins, veggies, and a tasty dip or sauce for a balanced and visually appealing lunch.

4. Cold Noodle Jars:

Layer cold noodles, shredded veggies, and a flavorful sauce in a jar. Enjoy a chilled noodle dish straight from the jar, perfect for a refreshing lunch on warm days.

5. Stuffed Pita Pockets:

Fill whole-grain pita pockets with a mixture of leftovers, add some fresh greens, and drizzle with your favorite dressing for a handheld and satisfying lunch.

6. Mini Veggie Skewers:

Thread bite-sized leftover vegetables onto skewers and pack them in your lunchbox. Dip them in a tasty sauce for a fun and interactive lunch option.

7. Hummus and Veggie Dippers:

Pack a container with hummus and an assortment of fresh vegetable sticks for a nutritious and easy-to-assemble lunch. Dip and enjoy!

Explore these lunchbox-friendly recipes and creative ways to repurpose leftovers to make your midday meals exciting and enjoyable.

Note: These ideas and recipes are designed to provide inspiration, and ingredient quantities can be adjusted based on personal preferences.

Chapter 6: Bonus Templates

- Weekly Meal Planner

- Shopping List Template

- Recipe Notes

- (Bonus) 2024 Monthly Planners

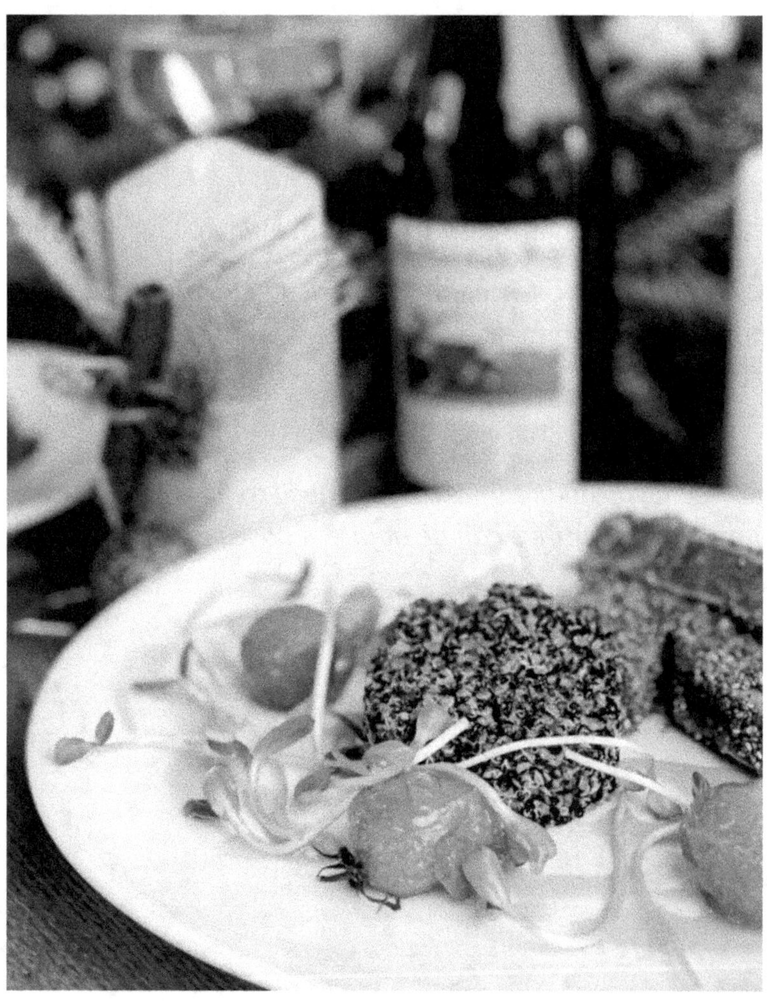

MEAL PLANNER

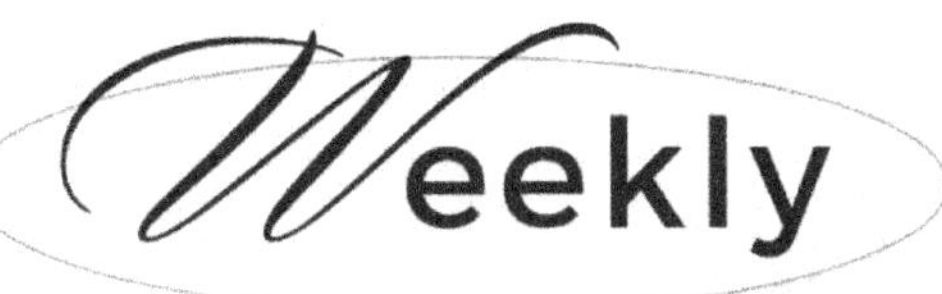

WEEK _______________   **MONTH** _______________

MONDAY

SATURDAY

TUESDAY

SUNDAY

WEDNESDAY

SHOPPING LIST

THURSDAY

FRIDAY

weekly
meal planner

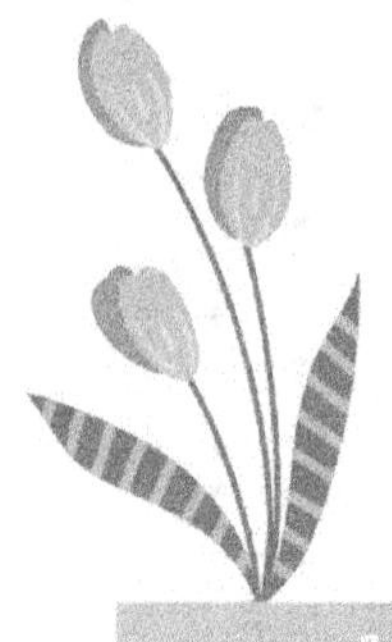

	BREAKFAST	LUNCH	DINNER	SNACKS
M				
T				
W				
T				
F				
S				
S				

WEEKLY SHOPPING LIST

DATE: ____

☑ OK   ☒ NOT AVAILABLE

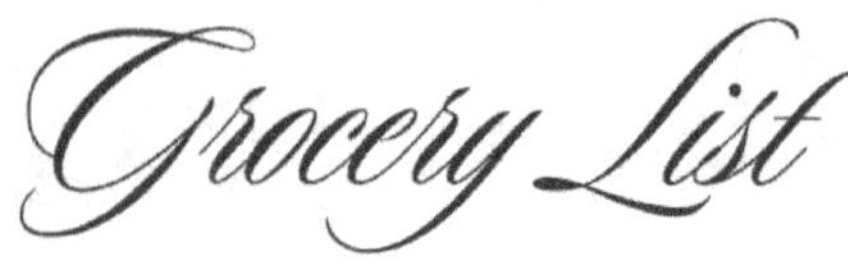

Grocery List

DATE: /   /

DAIRY:
○ __________
○ __________
○ __________
○ __________
○ __________
○ __________
○ __________
○ __________
○ __________
○ __________
○ __________
○ __________

MEAT & SEAFOOD:
○ __________
○ __________
○ __________
○ __________
○ __________
○ __________
○ __________
○ __________
○ __________
○ __________
○ __________
○ __________

FRUITS & VEGGIES:
○ __________
○ __________
○ __________
○ __________
○ __________
○ __________
○ __________
○ __________

BREAD & CEREAL:
○ __________
○ __________
○ __________
○ __________
○ __________

OTHERS:
○ __________
○ __________
○ __________
○ __________
○ __________
○ __________
○ __________
○ __________

FROZEN FOODS:
○ __________
○ __________
○ __________
○ __________
○ __________

CANNED GOODS:
○ __________
○ __________
○ __________
○ __________
○ __________

WHAT'S COOKING:
S __________
M __________
T __________
W __________
T __________
F __________
S __________

Recipe Card Planner

NAME OF RECIPE

DIFFICULTY

SERVES _______________

PREP TIME _______________

COOKING TEMP _______________

REVIEW ☆ ☆ ☆ ☆ ☆

◯ VEGETARIAN

◯ LOW CARB

◯ GLUTEN FREE

◯ DAIRY FREE

NOTES:

INGREDIENTS

METHOD

RECIPE CARD

INGREDIENTS:

DIRECTIONS:

Serves

prep

cook

Notes

01 JANUARY 2024

SUNDAY	MONDAY	TUESDAY	WEDNESDAY	THURSDAY	FRIDAY	SATURDAY
	1	2	3	4	5	6
7	8	9	10	11	12	13
14	15	16	17	18	19	20
21	22	23	24	25	26	27
28	29	30	31			

TO DO

NOTE

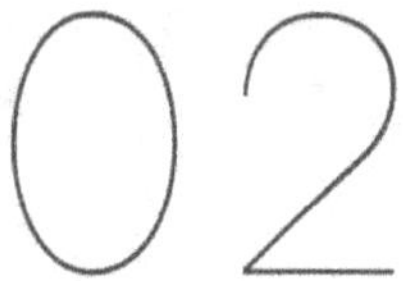

02

FEBRUARY
2024

SUNDAY	MONDAY	TUESDAY	WEDNESDAY	THURSDAY	FRIDAY	SATURDAY
				1	2	3
4	5	6	7	8	9	10
11	12	13	14	15	16	17
18	19	20	21	22	23	24
25	26	27	28	29		

TO DO

NOTE

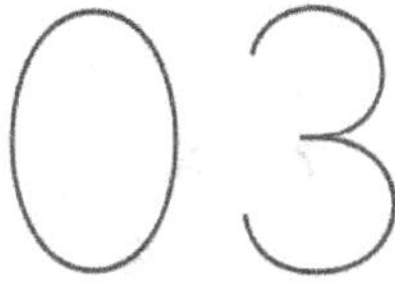

03

SUNDAY	MONDAY	TUESDAY	WEDNESDAY	THURSDAY	FRIDAY	SATURDAY
					1	2
3	4	5	6	7	8	9
10	11	12	13	14	15	16
17	18	19	20	21	22	23
24	25	26	27	28	29	30
31						

TO DO

NOTE

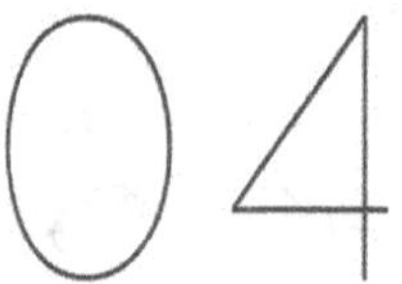

APRIL
2024

SUNDAY	MONDAY	TUESDAY	WEDNESDAY	THURSDAY	FRIDAY	SATURDAY
	1	2	3	4	5	6
7	8	9	10	11	12	13
14	15	16	17	18	19	20
21	22	23	24	25	26	27
28	29	30				

TO DO

NOTE

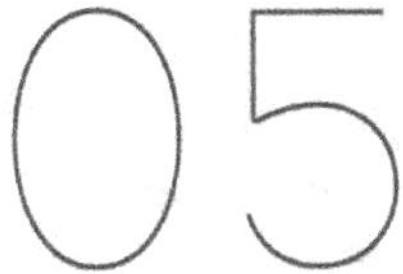

05

MAY
2024

SUNDAY	MONDAY	TUESDAY	WEDNESDAY	THURSDAY	FRIDAY	SATURDAY
			1	2	3	4
5	6	7	8	9	10	11
12	13	14	15	16	17	18
19	20	21	22	23	24	25
26	27	28	29	30	31	

TO DO

NOTE

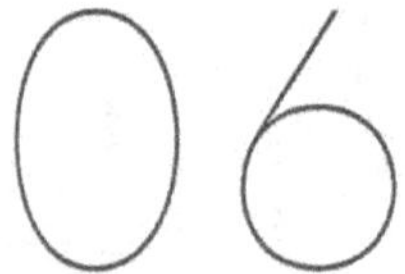

JUNE
2024

SUNDAY	MONDAY	TUESDAY	WEDNESDAY	THURSDAY	FRIDAY	SATURDAY
						1
2	3	4	5	6	7	8
9	10	11	12	13	14	15
16	17	18	19	20	21	22
23 / 30	24	25	26	27	28	29

TO DO

NOTE

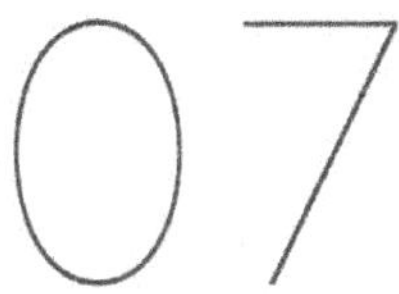

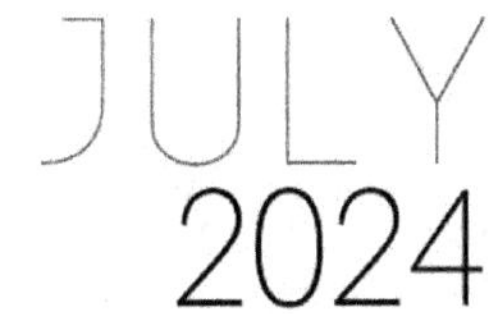

07

JULY
2024

SUNDAY	MONDAY	TUESDAY	WEDNESDAY	THURSDAY	FRIDAY	SATURDAY
	1	2	3	4	5	6
7	8	9	10	11	12	13
14	15	16	17	18	19	20
21	22	23	24	25	26	27
28	29	30	31			

TO DO

NOTE

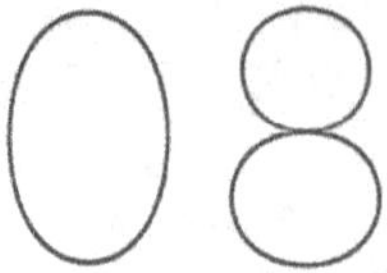

08

AUGUST
2024

SUNDAY	MONDAY	TUESDAY	WEDNESDAY	THURSDAY	FRIDAY	SATURDAY
				1	2	3
4	5	6	7	8	9	10
11	12	13	14	15	16	17
18	19	20	21	22	23	24
25	26	27	28	29	30	31

TO DO

NOTE

09 SEPTEMBER 2024

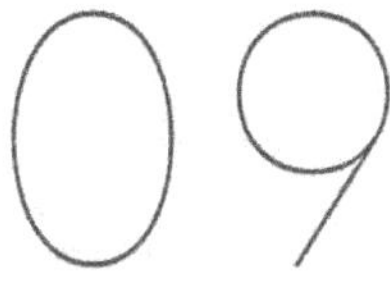

SUNDAY	MONDAY	TUESDAY	WEDNESDAY	THURSDAY	FRIDAY	SATURDAY
1	2	3	4	5	6	7
8	9	10	11	12	13	14
15	16	17	18	19	20	21
22	23	24	25	26	27	28
29	30					

TO DO

NOTE

10 OCTOBER 2024

SUNDAY	MONDAY	TUESDAY	WEDNESDAY	THURSDAY	FRIDAY	SATURDAY
		1	2	3	4	5
6	7	8	9	10	11	12
13	14	15	16	17	18	19
20	21	22	23	24	25	26
27	28	29	30	31		

TO DO

NOTE

11

NOVEMBER
2024

SUNDAY	MONDAY	TUESDAY	WEDNESDAY	THURSDAY	FRIDAY	SATURDAY
					1	2
3	4	5	6	7	8	9
10	11	12	13	14	15	16
17	18	19	20	21	22	23
24	25	26	27	28	29	30

TO DO

NOTE

12

SUNDAY	MONDAY	TUESDAY	WEDNESDAY	THURSDAY	FRIDAY	SATURDAY
1	2	3	4	5	6	7
8	9	10	11	12	13	14
15	16	17	18	19	20	21
22	23	24	25	26	27	28
29	30	31				

TO DO

NOTE

Chapter 7: Tips for Dining Out on Weekends

- Making Healthy Choices

- Restaurant Survival Guide

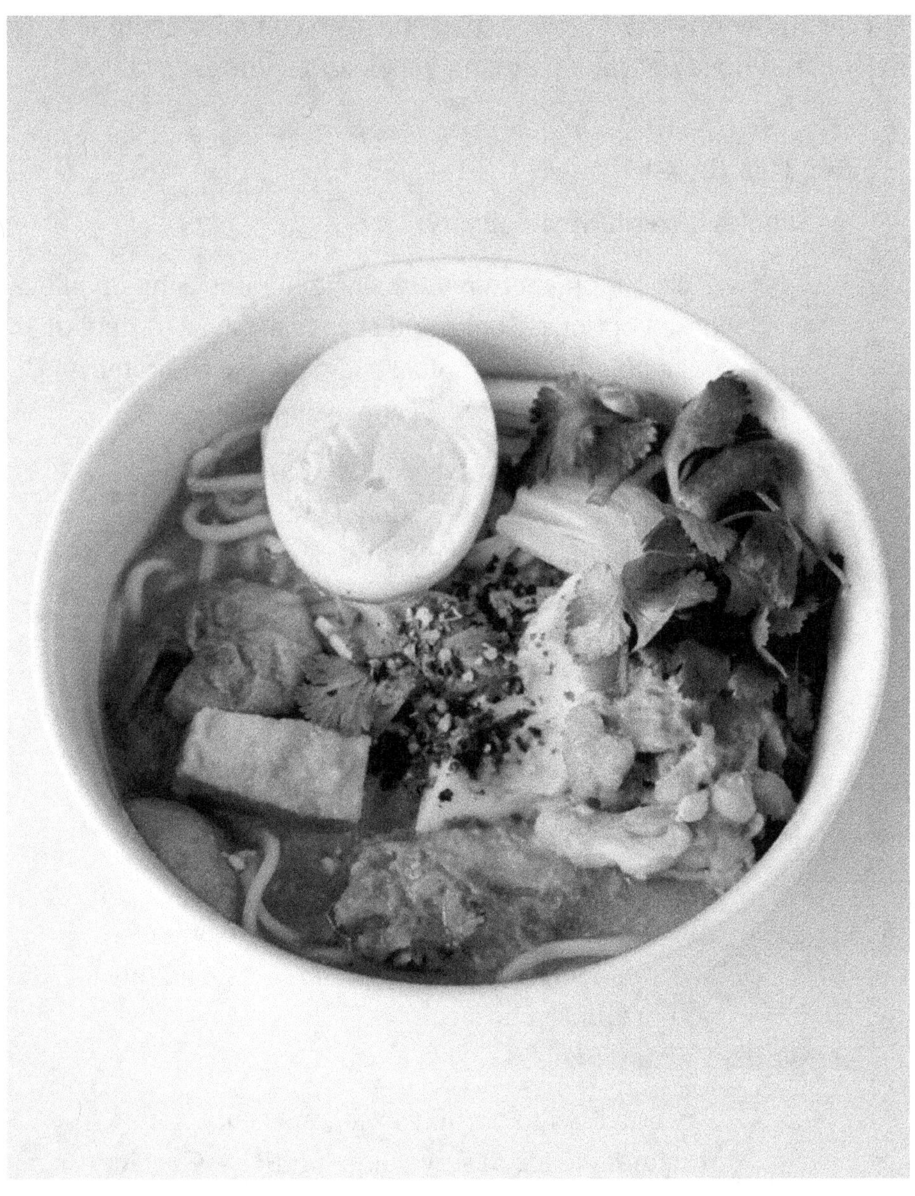

Chapter 7: Tips for Dining Out on Weekends

Dining out on weekends can be a delightful experience, and this chapter is here to guide you in making healthy choices and navigating restaurant menus with confidence. Whether you're meeting friends, celebrating special occasions, or simply taking a break from the kitchen, these tips will help you maintain your commitment to a plant-based lifestyle while enjoying the pleasures of restaurant dining.

Making Healthy Choices

1. **Scan the Menu Strategically:**

   - Take a moment to review the menu, focusing on plant-based options. Look for dishes featuring a variety of vegetables, whole grains, and plant-based proteins.

2. **Opt for Grilled or Roasted Preparations:**

   - Choose dishes that are grilled, roasted, or baked instead of fried. These cooking methods enhance flavors without excessive use of oil and contribute to a healthier dining experience.

3. **Build Your Own Plate:**

   - Many restaurants offer customizable options. Take advantage of this by building your own plate with a mix of plant-based proteins, vegetables, and grains.

4. **Inquire about Ingredient Substitutions:**

   - Don't hesitate to ask if certain ingredients can be substituted or omitted. Restaurants are often accommodating to dietary preferences, and this allows you to tailor your meal.

5. **Watch Portion Sizes:**

   - Pay attention to portion sizes, especially if the restaurant tends to serve large portions. Consider sharing dishes or opting for appetizers to control the quantity of food.

6. **Balance Your Plate:**

   - Aim for a balanced plate with a variety of colors and textures. Include a mix of leafy greens, vibrant vegetables, and protein sources to ensure a well-rounded and satisfying meal.

Restaurant Survival Guide

1. **Communicate Your Dietary Preferences:**

   - When you arrive at the restaurant, don't hesitate to communicate your dietary preferences to the server. They can provide insights into the menu and guide you towards suitable options.

2. **Ask for Modifications:**

   - If a dish almost fits your preferences but needs a tweak, ask for modifications. Restaurants are often willing to adjust preparations to accommodate dietary needs.

3. **Be Mindful of Sauces and Dressings:**

   - Sauces and dressings can add hidden calories and ingredients. Request them on the side or ask for lighter alternatives to control the flavor profile of your meal.

4. **Hydrate Wisely:**

   - Make water your primary beverage choice. If you opt for alcoholic beverages, do so in moderation, and consider lower-calorie options like wine or light beer.

5. **Savor Mindfully:**

   - Enjoy your meal slowly, savoring each bite. This not only enhances your dining experience but also allows your body to signal fullness more effectively.

6. **Plan Ahead for Dessert:**

- If you're planning to indulge in dessert, be mindful of your choices earlier in the meal. Consider sharing a dessert or opting for fruit-based options.

By incorporating these tips, you can dine out with confidence, enjoy delicious plant-based meals, and make the most of your weekend dining experiences.

Note: These tips are designed to provide guidance, and individuals can tailor them to their preferences and dietary needs.

Conclusion

- Recap of Benefits

- Encouragement for a Healthier Lifestyle

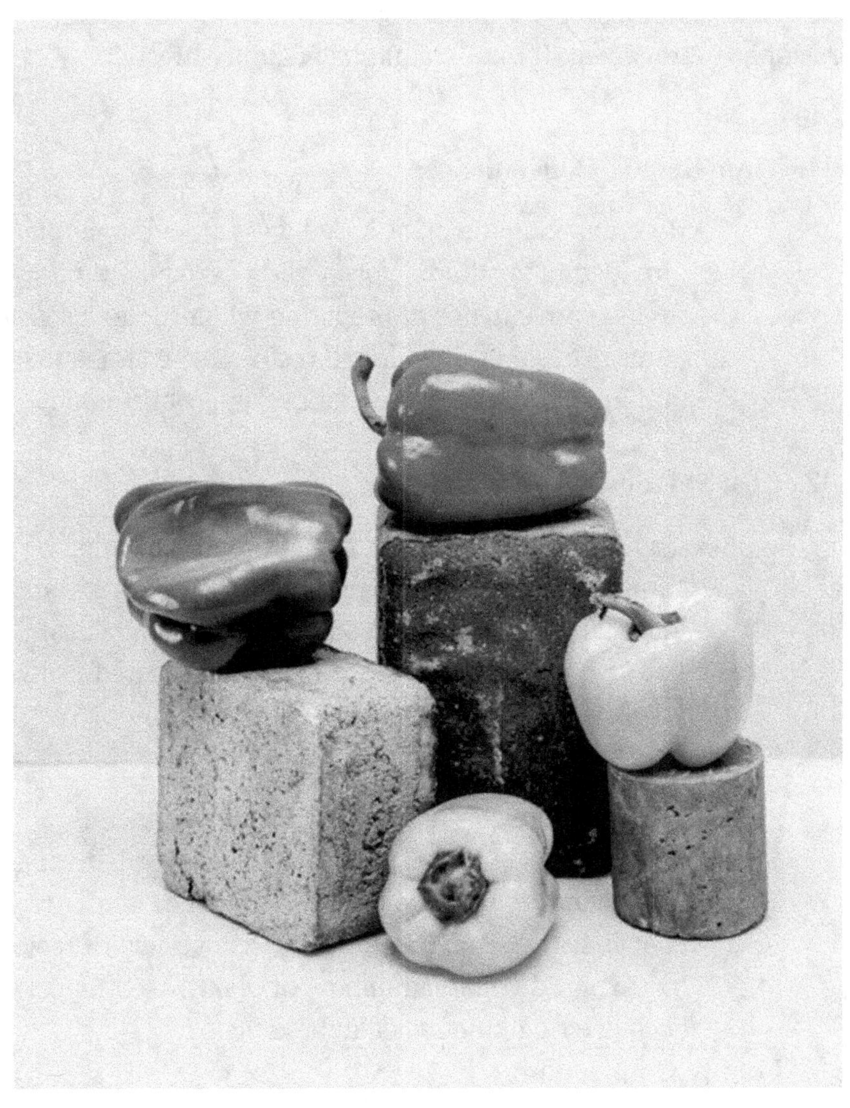

Conclusion

Congratulations on completing the journey through "Weeknight Vegan & Vegetarian Delights: A Month of Healthy Dinners for Busy Lives." In this concluding chapter, let's recap the benefits you've gained from adopting a plant-based approach, and I'll share some words of encouragement for maintaining a healthier lifestyle.

Recap of Benefits

1. **Time-Saving Convenience:**

   - By embracing the plant-based weeknight dinner plans provided in this book, you've discovered the time-saving convenience of preparing wholesome meals at home. The carefully curated recipes have aimed to minimize cooking time without compromising on flavor and nutrition.

2. **Cost Savings:**

   - Cooking at home often translates to cost savings compared to dining out regularly. By planning your meals and utilizing leftovers for next-day lunches, you've not only saved money but also ensured that your plant-based journey is budget-friendly.

3. **Nutritional Enrichment:**

   - Plant-based meals are rich in vitamins, minerals, and fiber. Throughout this book, you've explored diverse ingredients, ensuring a broad spectrum of nutrients that contribute to overall well-being. The variety of recipes has exposed you to a rainbow of plant-based foods, each offering unique health benefits.

4. **Family Connection:**

   - The small family-sized servings provided in the meal plans encourage shared dining experiences. Whether it's enjoying a cozy dinner together or bringing leftovers for lunch, these moments foster family connections and provide a shared appreciation for plant-based goodness.

5. **Environmental Impact:**

   - By choosing plant-based meals, you've contributed to a positive environmental impact. Plant-based diets generally have a lower carbon footprint compared to animal-based diets, making your culinary choices part of a broader commitment to sustainability.

Encouragement for a Healthier Lifestyle

1. **Celebrate Your Achievements:**

   - Take a moment to celebrate your achievements on this plant-based journey. Whether you've tried new ingredients, discovered a favorite recipe, or consistently cooked at home, every step is a victory toward a healthier lifestyle.

2. **Flexibility and Exploration:**

   - Remember that plant-based eating is not a rigid set of rules but a flexible and exploratory adventure. Feel free to experiment with flavors, modify recipes to suit your taste, and continuously explore the world of plant-based cuisine.

3. **Listen to Your Body:**

   - Pay attention to how your body responds to plant-based meals. Notice changes in energy levels, digestion, and overall well-being. Adjust your approach based on what makes you feel your best.

4. **Community Support:**

   - Connect with the plant-based community for support and inspiration. Share your experiences, seek advice, and celebrate successes together. Having a supportive community can make the journey more enjoyable and sustainable.

5. **Mindful Eating Practices:**

   - Practice mindful eating by savoring each bite, appreciating the flavors and textures of your meals. Mindful eating not only enhances your dining experience but also fosters a healthier relationship with food.

As you conclude this book, know that you hold the power to shape your health and well-being through the choices you make in the kitchen. Whether you continue on a fully plant-based path or incorporate more plant-centric meals into your routine, the positive impact on your health and the environment is substantial. Here's to your continued success in creating delicious, nourishing, and sustainable meals for yourself and your loved ones.

Appendix

- Ingredient Substitution Guide

- Metric Conversion Chart

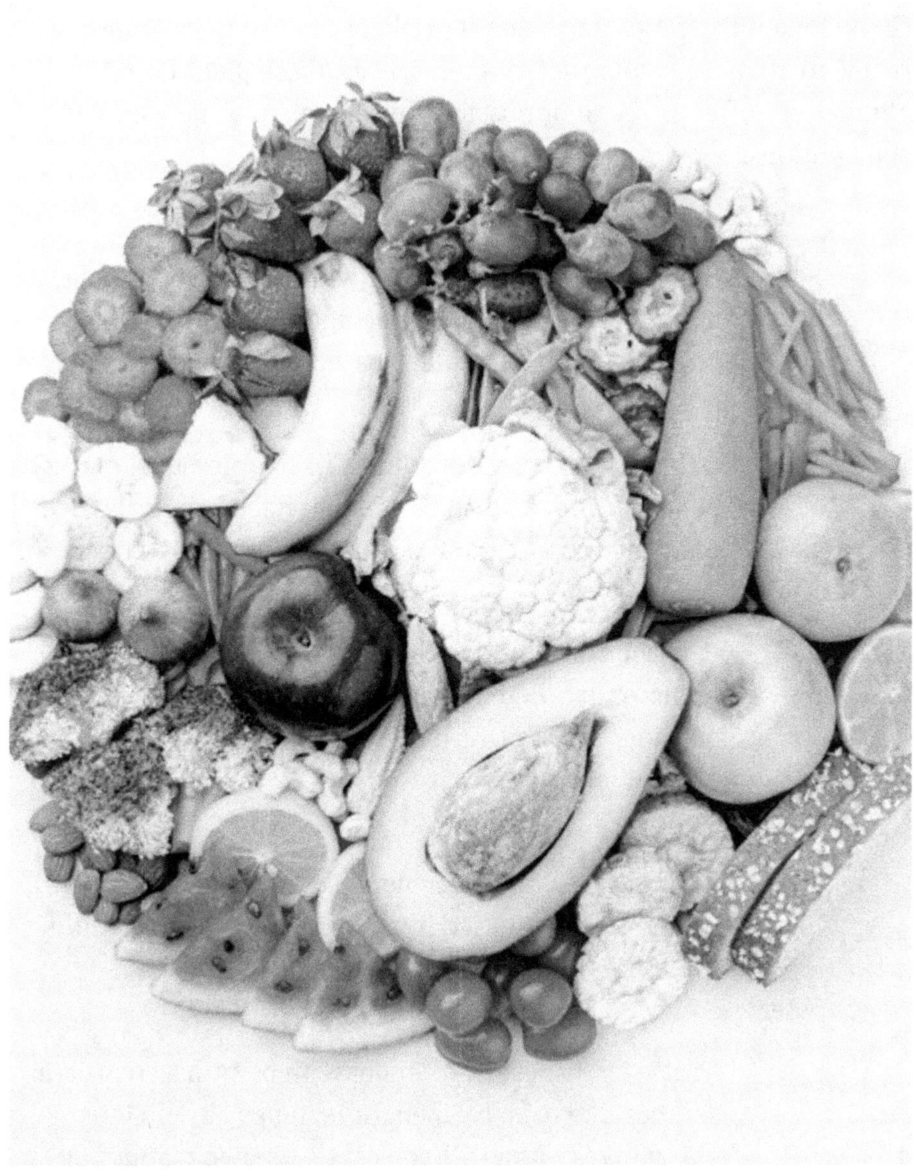

Appendix

Plant-Based Ingredient Substitution Guide

In the world of plant-based cooking, adaptability is key, and this Ingredient Substitution Guide is here to empower you in navigating the diverse landscape of plant-centric culinary creations. Whether you find yourself missing a particular ingredient or wish to customize a recipe to align with your dietary preferences, these plant-based alternatives offer a wealth of possibilities. Here are some valuable substitutions:

1. **Flour:**

   - Substitute all-purpose flour with whole wheat flour, almond flour, or gluten-free options like rice flour or chickpea flour for a plant-based twist.

2. **Eggs:**

   - In baking, explore substitutes like applesauce, mashed bananas, yogurt, or flaxseed gel. Each brings its own unique texture and flavor to your plant-based treats.

3. **Dairy:**

   - Replace dairy milk with plant-based alternatives such as almond milk, coconut milk, or soy milk. For butter, consider using plant-based oils like olive oil or coconut oil.

4. **Sugar:**

   - Embrace natural sweeteners like maple syrup, agave nectar, or plant-based honey alternatives as substitutes for white or brown sugar.

5. **Meat:**

   - In savory dishes, experiment with plant-based protein sources like tofu, tempeh, or legumes as delicious alternatives to meat. Each offers its own distinct texture and flavor.

6. **Cheese:**

> ⌄ Opt for nutritional yeast, cashew cream, or vegan cheese options as dairy-free alternatives for recipes that call for cheese.

Remember, the world of plant-based substitutions is vast, and the best choice often depends on the specific dish you're preparing. Allow this guide to be your companion in creating flavorful and satisfying plant-based meals tailored to your taste preferences and dietary needs.

Metric Conversion Chart

Cooking is a universal language, and the Metric Conversion Chart provided here is your guide to a seamless culinary experience, especially if you prefer or are accustomed to metric measurements. Here's a quick reference:

- ⌄ **Volume:**

  - ⌄ 1 cup ≈ 240 milliliters
  - ⌄ 1 tablespoon ≈ 15 milliliters
  - ⌄ 1 teaspoon ≈ 5 milliliters

- ⌄ **Weight:**

  - ⌄ 1 pound ≈ 454 grams
  - ⌄ 1 ounce ≈ 28 grams

- ⌄ **Temperature:**

  - ⌄ 350°F ≈ 180°C
  - ⌄ 375°F ≈ 190°C
  - ⌄ 400°F ≈ 200°C

May this guide serve as your companion, providing valuable insights into plant-based substitutions and metric conversions, enriching your plant-based culinary journey. Happy cooking!

Encouragement

- Encouragement from the author

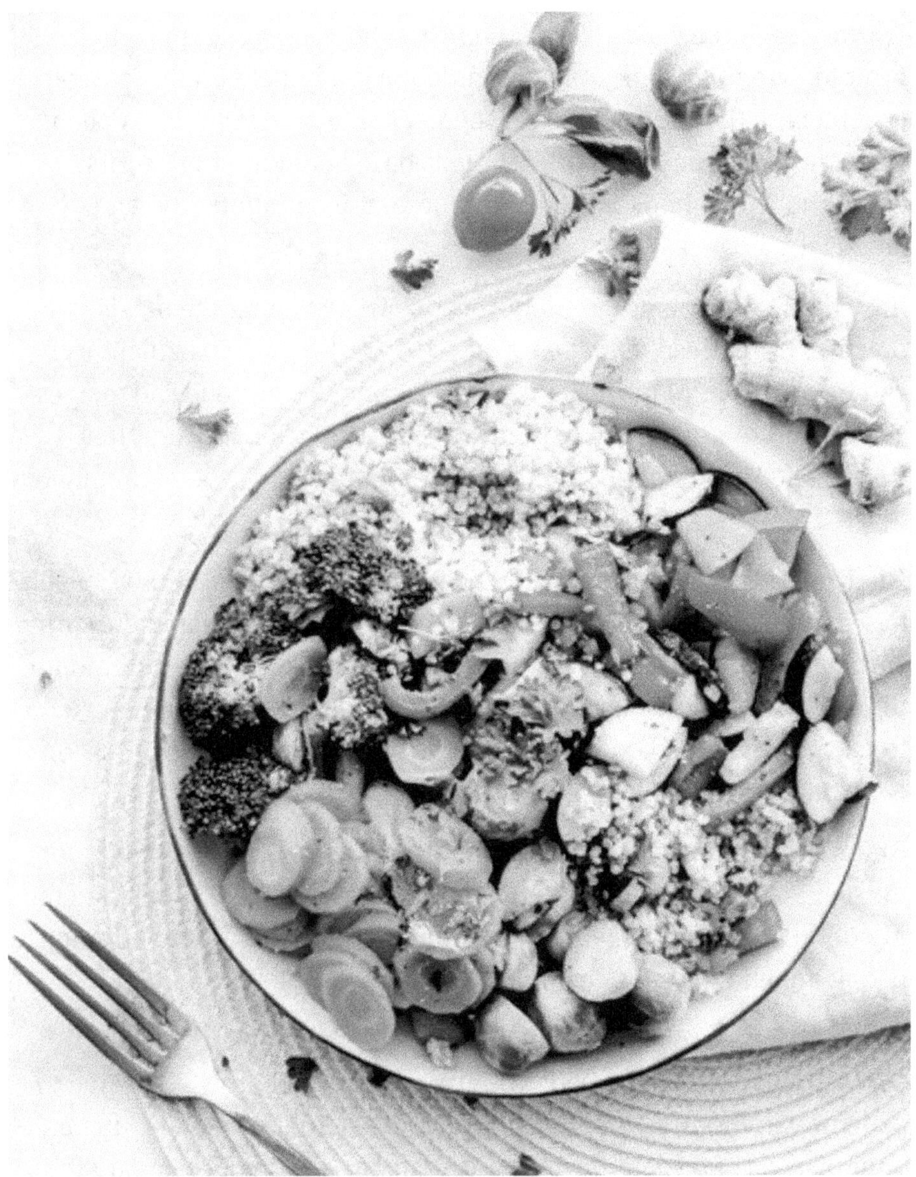

Encouragement from the Author

Dear Reader,

As you reach the end of "Weeknight Vegan & Vegetarian Delights," I want to extend my sincerest gratitude for joining me on this culinary adventure. Whether you're a seasoned chef, a novice in the kitchen, or someone exploring the world of plant-based cooking for the first time, I hope this book has been a source of inspiration, joy, and practical guidance.

Embarking on a plant-based journey is not just about the meals you prepare; it's a lifestyle that encompasses well-being, sustainability, and the pleasure of savoring delicious, nourishing food. The recipes shared in these pages are crafted with care, focusing on simplicity, flavor, and the joy of creating wholesome meals for yourself and your loved ones.

Remember that every step you take toward incorporating more plant-based meals into your routine is a step toward a healthier and more sustainable lifestyle. Whether you choose to dive into the full month of meal plans or pick and choose recipes that speak to you, the goal is to make plant-based cooking a delightful and accessible part of your everyday life.

Embrace the journey with an open heart and a willingness to explore the abundance of flavors that the plant kingdom offers. Celebrate the joy of creating meals that not only nourish your body but also bring people together around the dinner table.

If you encounter challenges along the way, remember that every cooking experience is an opportunity to learn and grow. Feel free to experiment, modify, and make these recipes your own. The kitchen is your canvas, and each meal is a masterpiece waiting to be crafted.

Thank you for allowing me to be a part of your culinary adventure. May your kitchen be filled with the aromas of wholesome ingredients, and may each bite bring you closer to a healthier and more vibrant you.

Wishing you many delicious moments,

Jenny Koo

Happy Cooking!

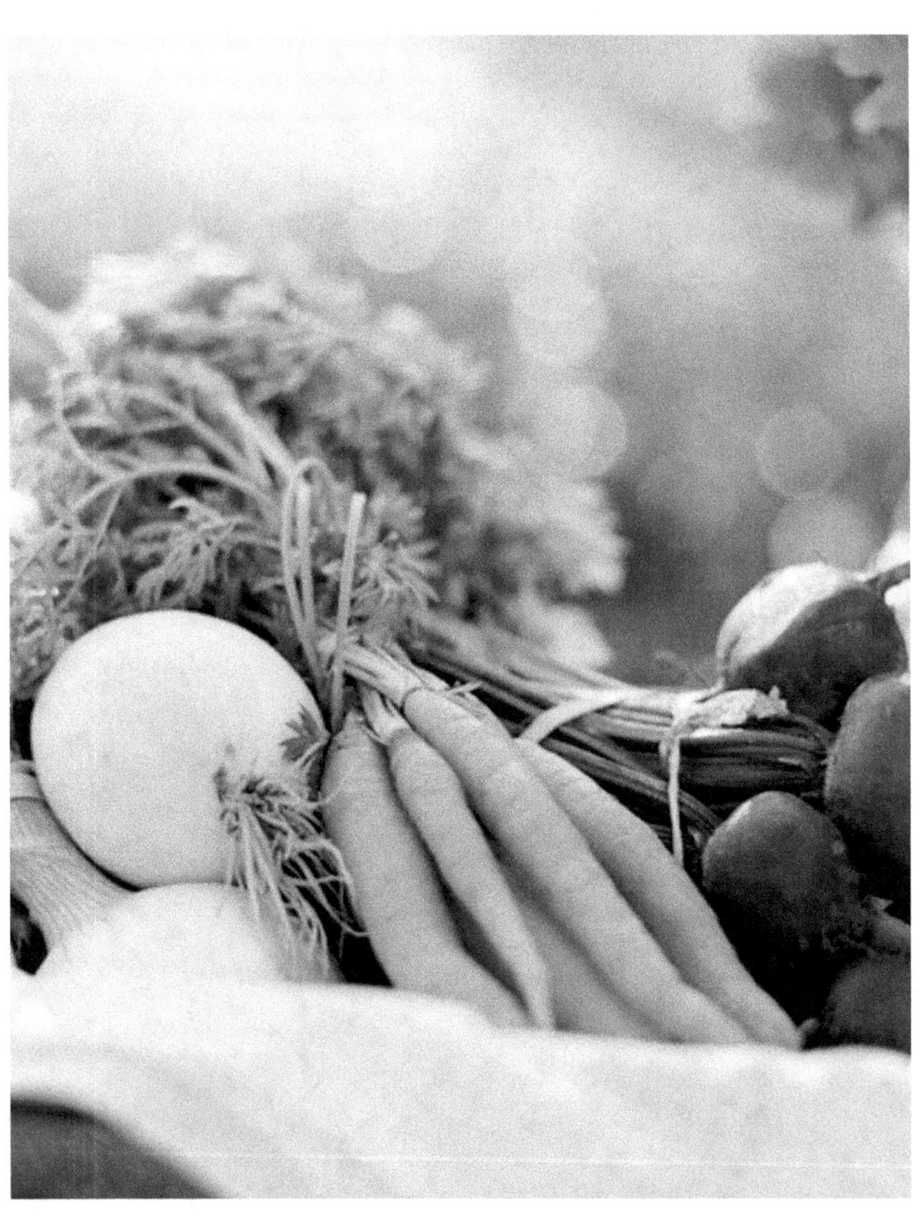

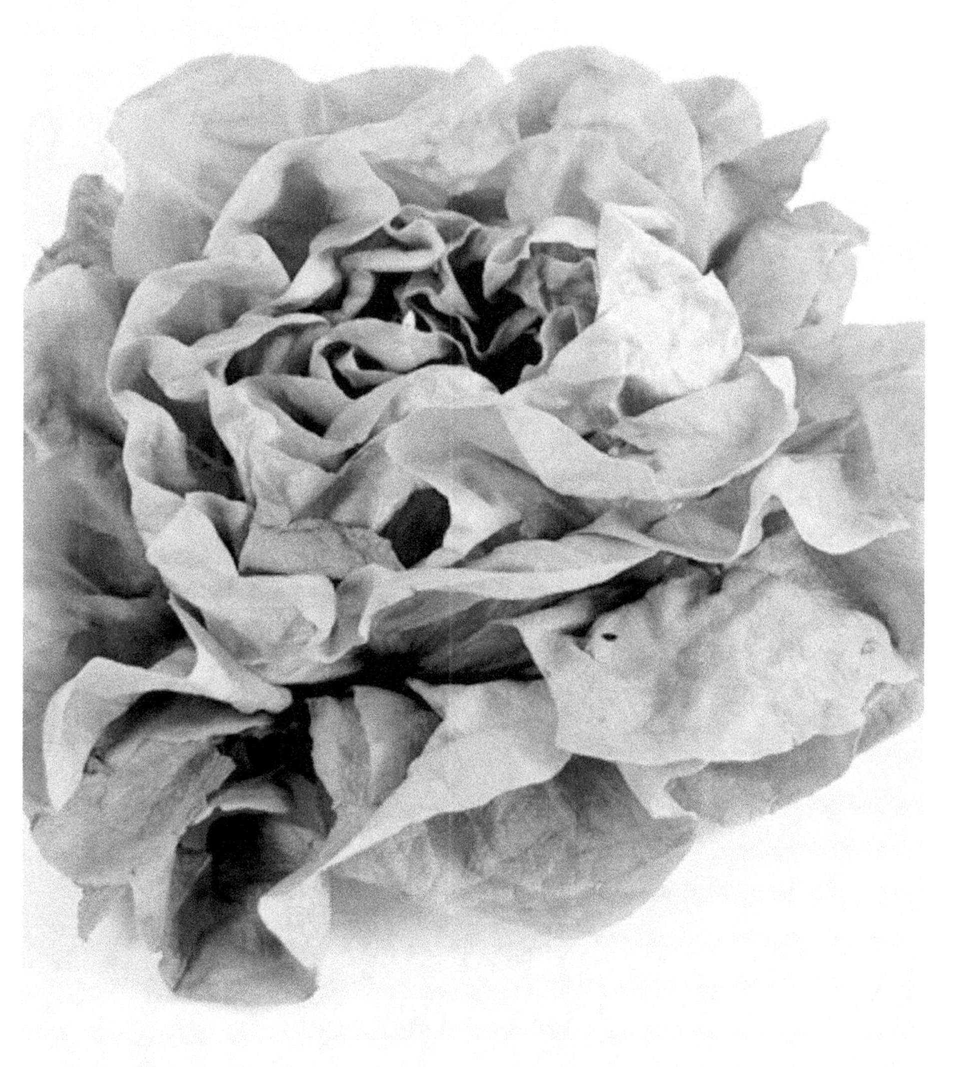

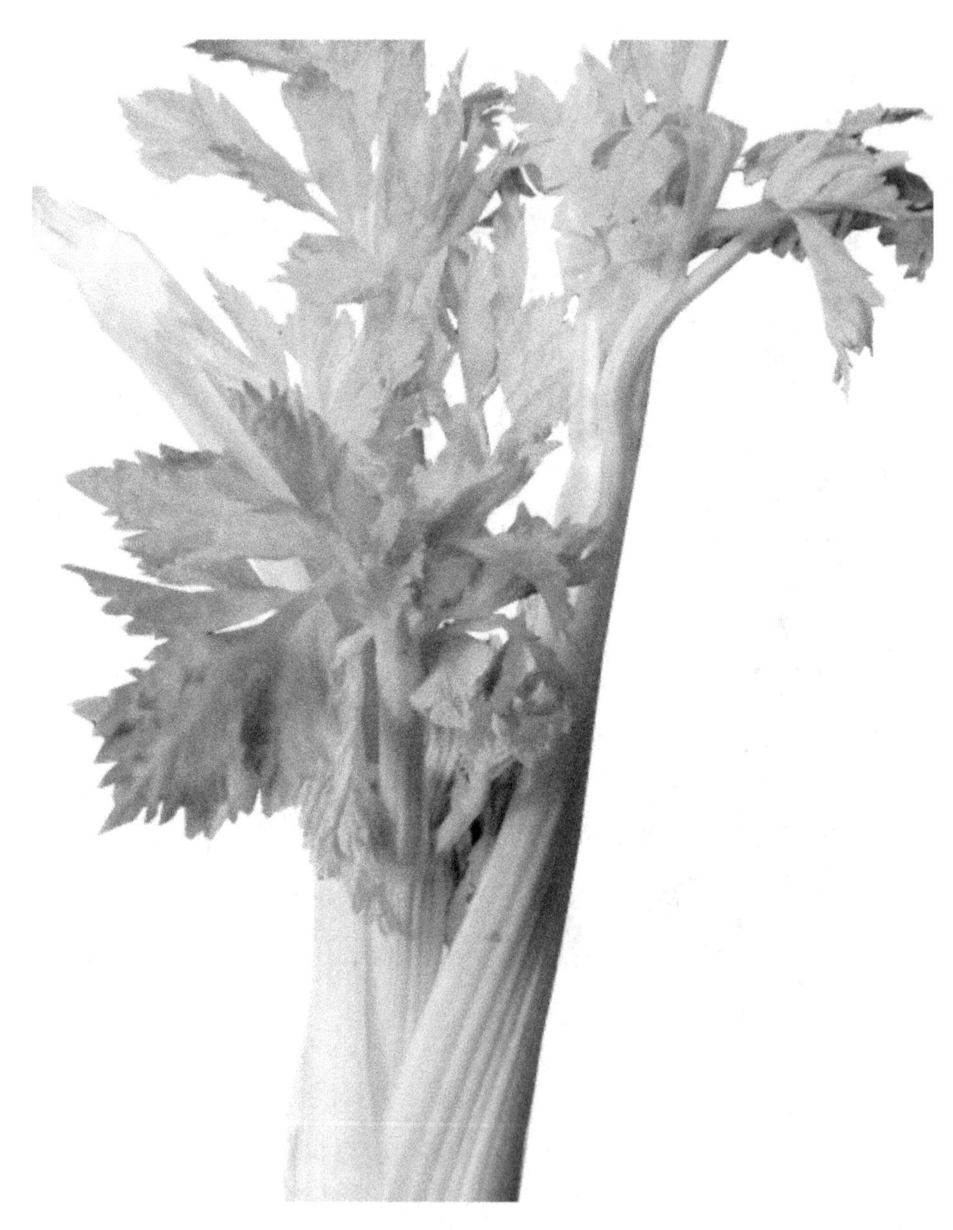

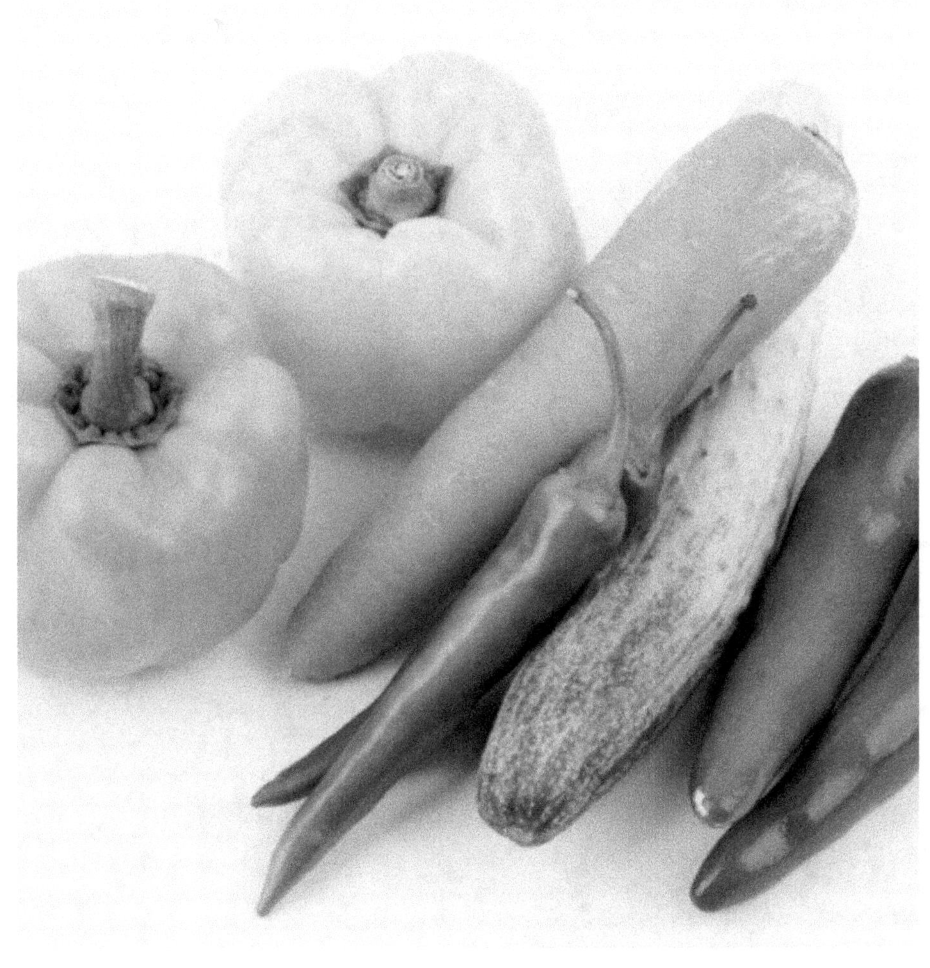

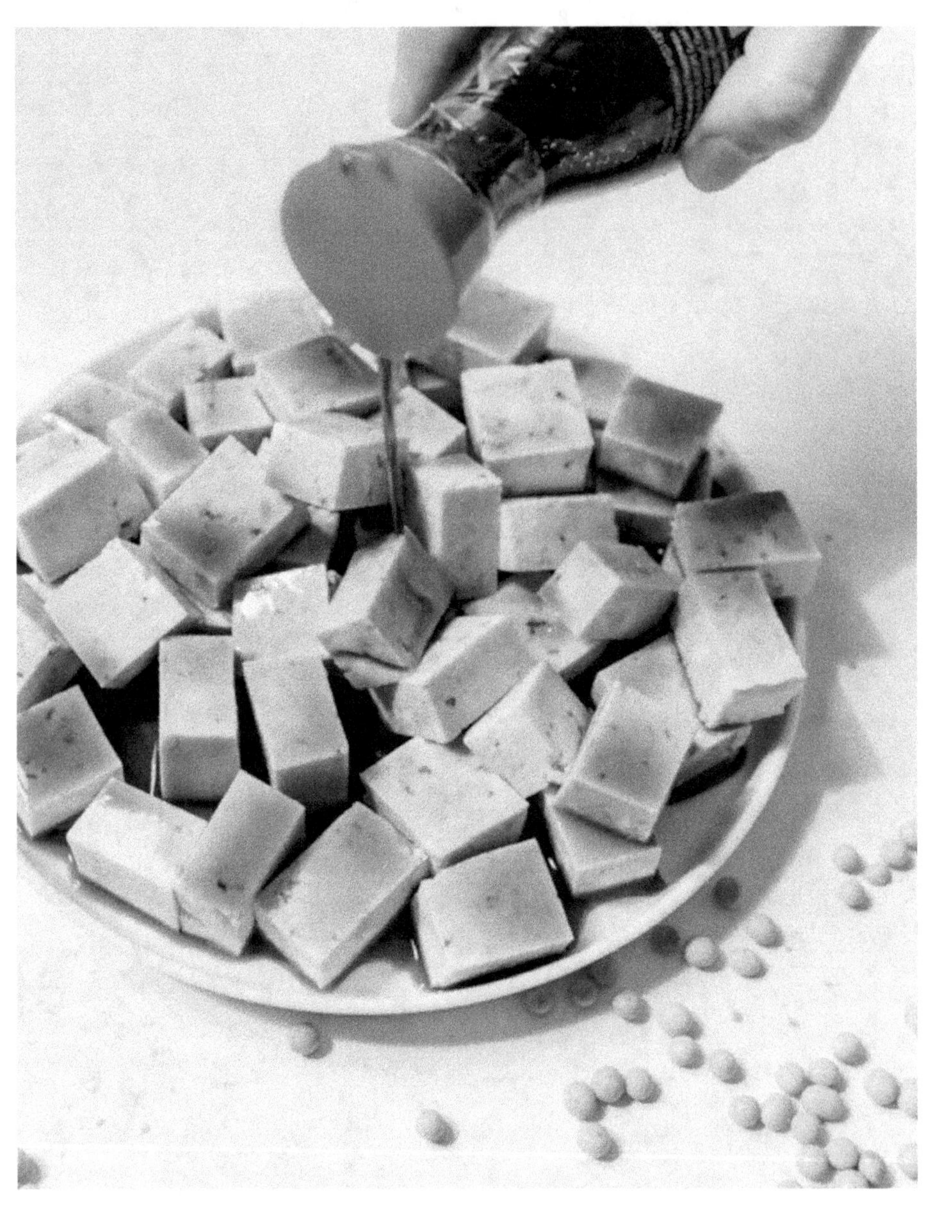